Midwifery FOR EXPECTANT PARENTS

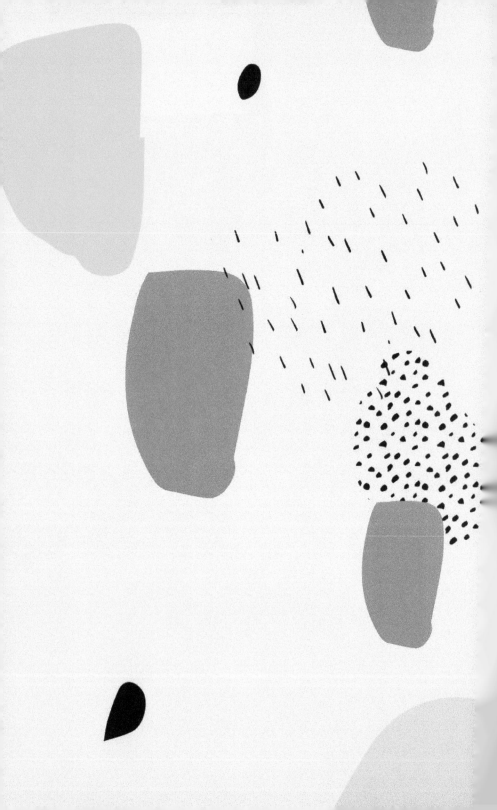

Midwifery

FOR EXPECTANT PARENTS

A Modern Guide to Choosing the Birth That's Right for You

AUBRE TOMPKINS, CNM

ROCKRIDGE PRESS

Interior and Cover Designer: Julie Schrader
Art Producer: Sara Feinstein
Editor: Lauren O'Neal
Production Editor: Mia Moran
Illustrations used under license from iStock.com, pp. 5, 22, 33, 38, 57, 73, 87, 113, 115, 125, 139, 151; Shutterstock.com, pp. 47, 51, 81; All other illustrations used under license from © Emma Make/Creative Market.
Photography © Chelsea Victoria/Stocksy, p. 15; Jakob Lagerstedt/Stocksy, p. 43; Lea Csontos/Stocksy, p. 97, iStock.com, pp. 152
Author photo courtesy of © Lindsey Eden
ISBN: Print 978-1-64739-048-8 | eBook 978-1-64739-049-5
R0

To family: my own dear family,
without whom I could not do this work,
and the wonderful families that have allowed
me to serve them as a midwife.

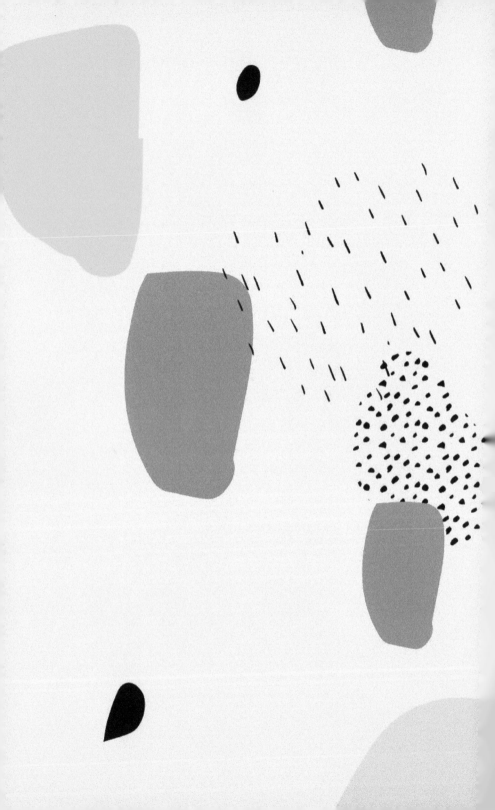

Contents

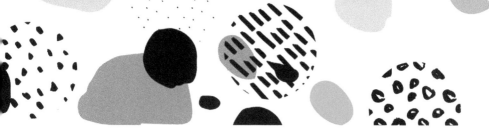

Introduction

LET ME START OFF by welcoming you to this journey of pregnancy and parenthood! It's an exciting season that can also, at times, feel overwhelming. I hope the words found in these pages can alleviate some of your anxiety and help you feel educated and empowered about your choices. Whether you're already pregnant or trying to conceive, it's never too early to know your choices and educate yourself. As a pregnant person, you'll need to make many decisions about your care. It is my goal to offer you the information and support necessary to make the best choices for you and your family.

I have been immersed in the world of maternity care for well over 20 years—first as a mother myself, then as a registered nurse, and finally as a midwife. When I was pregnant with my first child, I was not yet a nurse and truly knew next to nothing about pregnancy or birth. It was through the support of a wonderful hospital-based midwifery group that I found the knowledge and strength to begin my parenting journey. The care I received empowered me and fed my soul. It also awakened in me a desire to become a midwife myself.

I decided that I would become a certified nurse midwife (CNM), but the first step was to become a registered nurse (RN). As an RN, I started working in a busy hospital and spent time on the labor floor, in the postpartum unit and well-baby nursery, and in the neonatal intensive care unit (NICU). I also started working at a freestanding birth

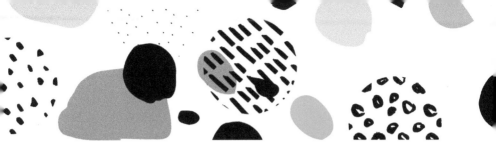

center—a facility not attached to a hospital where families go to have their babies. At the birth center, I attended births and ran baby-care and breastfeeding education programs. Eventually, I went on to midwifery school, and since then, I've worked in both freestanding birth centers and a hospital practice. I chose to give birth to my youngest child at home with a midwife and my family at my side, and I had an amazingly powerful experience.

The work of midwifery is incredibly fulfilling. I view it as a blessing to be invited into this most intimate space. I also view it as an immeasurable responsibility, not to be taken lightly. Birth truly is an everyday miracle. That it happens every minute of every day around the globe doesn't make it less miraculous—it makes it more human, as we are all touched by our own births and those of the people around us.

As a midwife, it's my job to oversee the health and safety of my clients as well as to provide emotional and psychological support along the way. In a sense, this book allows me to offer my midwifery services to more folks than I ever could in person. I am honored to be able to share my experience with you and your family. So please feel free to sit back, sip a cup of warm herbal tea, put your feet up, and allow me to join you on this journey.

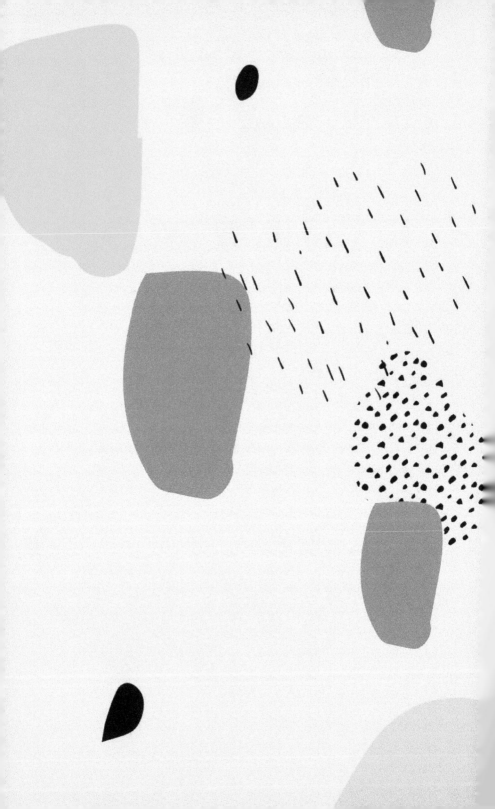

CHAPTER 1

All about Midwifery

Midwives have been around nearly as long as human beings have been giving birth. Over the centuries, the word "midwife" has taken on many meanings, from a folk healer to a type of physician to the modern definition: a trained and certified professional who specializes in the care of women and newborns during pregnancy and childbirth. If you're new to midwifery (or even if you're not), there can be lot to learn, and it can feel complicated. This chapter will give you an over-view of what midwifery is and the benefits of choosing midwifery care.

Midwifery through the Ages

Choosing to work with a midwife means joining a tradition that stretches back millennia and spans the globe. Though reading about the history of that tradition isn't a requirement for working with a midwife, learning the roots of the practice can help you better understand the wealth of information, knowledge, and experience that midwifery brings to your care.

Midwifery is a tradition that was historically handed down from practitioner to practitioner based on a combination of hands-on learning and oral transfer of knowledge. It was also traditionally only practiced by women. Since history has been written almost entirely from a male perspective, midwifery was often not well documented in the medical literature or cultural writings of any given era. It is clear, though, that midwives have always been present to guard the threshold of life.

Midwives appear in ancient Egyptian medical texts and art. There are "figure vessels" depicting midwives, and ancient Egyptian images of childbirth typically depicted women giving birth surrounded by other women and female deities. In ancient Greek and Roman writings, we find lengthy descriptions of midwives and the work they do—some of it not very different from the work midwives practice today. For example, an ancient Greek instruction manual for midwives, written by Soranus of Ephesus, included references to the "midwife's chair," which allowed a woman to give birth in an upright position with midwives beside her to offer support and guidance. Very similar birthing stools are still used by midwives today and are a great example of how midwifery utilizes traditions that have been handed down through the centuries while also folding in new scientific information.

The Bible references midwifery multiple times, such as in Exodus 1:15–21, when the king of Egypt orders midwives who attend the births of Hebrew families to immediately put all male babies to death. In an act of bravery and defiance, the midwives refuse to do so and let the children live.

Though midwives faced challenges throughout history, their difficulties increased as societies' attitudes toward women changed. During the Middle Ages in Europe, there was a widespread effort by the Catholic church to associate midwives with witchcraft and devil worship, which may have stemmed in part from the fact that many midwives were also healers and herbalists who had knowledge of women's health and the reproductive process. A "witch-hunting" text from the era claimed that midwives "surpass all others in wickedness." It is estimated that up to 250,000 people were executed as witches between 1300 and 1500 and that up to 85 percent of these people were women who were also accused of midwifery.

And it wasn't only happening in Europe—around the globe, midwives were targeted by societies that were increasing their efforts to control and objectify women's bodies. In China, for example, midwives were long an integral part of the health care system, providing primary care to women in their childbearing year (the months comprising pregnancy, birth, and the postpartum period). But starting in the late 1200s, they were pushed out in favor of the male-dominated medical system, which wanted to have more control over the practice of gynecology. In China today, midwives are still working to regain a foothold in providing care for families.

However, something very interesting happened in Europe after the Middle Ages. Midwifery was able to reestablish itself and become an integrated and respected part of the European health care system.

Modern Midwifery

Modern midwifery has grown and developed as our scientific understanding of the human body has expanded. It has also managed to hold true to its roots in supporting families and honoring the individual. Midwifery looks at the female body through a holistic lens of wellness and supports clients in making informed choices throughout their pregnancy, labor, birth, and beyond. It understands that the pregnant person is the expert on their own body and encourages them to become educated and empowered in the process.

In fact, the word "midwife" comes from a Middle English word meaning "with-woman." This etymology exemplifies one of midwifery's strongest tenets: We walk *with* our clients, alongside them, neither in front of nor behind them in stature. Yes, we have years of training and study that we bring along, but pregnant people have knowledge about their own bodies and needs that is always equal to our own. No one is more of an expert on your individual body than you. This focus on centering the pregnant person, coupled with the understanding of modern science and medicine, is one factor that sets midwifery apart from other birthing practices currently in use.

For many people, the word "midwife" may conjure up images of matronly women in long, flowing skirts and sandals, surrounded by clouds of patchouli and wearing a lot of crystals. To be sure, this type of midwife does exist. But a midwife may just as often be Harvard-educated and have a PhD in research or public health. And, though the vast majority of practitioners are women, midwives can also be men! Families come in all shapes and sizes, from all cultures and backgrounds, and so do midwives.

While times were tough for midwives in the Middle Ages, the practice slowly began to regain its footing in many countries. Today, in Norway, Sweden, France, the Netherlands, and the UK, midwives attend the majority of births. In these countries, pregnant people start with a midwife by default and only use a physician if their pregnancy becomes high-risk. Other countries, like Japan, also have high rates of midwife-attended births.

In the United States, midwives attend far fewer births—currently, the rate hovers at around 10 percent. Sadly, the United States spends the most money on maternity care but has the worst outcomes of any developed nation.

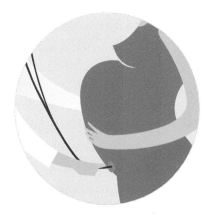

Midwifery in the United States

Prior to the forced colonization of the North American continent, the land was inhabited by indigenous people and cultures with rich histories spanning centuries. These nations had their own knowledge and traditions around birth, with midwives who practiced these skills. This must be acknowledged and recognized. But as a non–Native American, I'm not privy to these stories and practices, which must be told by the members of these nations in the settings they deem appropriate. As this book is not capable of telling the story of indigenous midwifery, it will instead focus on the midwifery brought to the United States from elsewhere.

When early European colonists arrived in North America, they brought with them their own health care traditions, practices, and providers. Some of these were, of course, midwives, who were an integral part of the community. In the South, African midwives who had been ripped from their homes and forced into slavery also brought their practices. Prior to emancipation, these midwives served the majority of both white and black Southern women. Even after emancipation, these midwives continued to serve poor black and white women. They are often referred to as "grand midwives" and were instrumental in keeping the threads of midwifery intact in our country, both by continuing the hands-on practice and by passing on the knowledge.

This midwifery tradition carried on until the late 1800s, when the modern American medical system began to take hold. As the number of medical-training institutions, hospitals, and clinics in the United States began to increase, so did the number of new physicians. These physicians, who needed patients to establish their own practices, encouraged pregnant women to work with them instead of midwives and began an active campaign against midwifery.

They painted midwifery as a backward, outdated, dangerous practice offered by dirty and uneducated women. Books, newspaper articles, and ads in prominent women's magazines of the day touted technology and medicalization over traditional knowledge. By the turn of the 20th century, the percentage of midwifery-attended births in the United States had declined from nearly 100 percent to only about 50 percent.

The medical establishment's efforts to discredit midwives continued into the 20th century. Midwifery was not recognized as a valid educational path, and women were denied entry into medical schools. Around 1910, the American Medical Association launched a campaign to erase midwifery. Over the course of the ensuing decades, this campaign was nearly successful in wiping out American midwifery. By the 1930s, midwife-attended births had fallen to 15 percent, and by the turn of the 21st century, well over 90 percent of births were attended by physicians. Interestingly, during this decline in midwifery, rates of poor outcomes for women and babies increased.

Slowly and tenaciously, midwives have been working to regain respect and acceptance in the United States. While around 10 percent of US births are attended by midwives, in some states, that number is much higher—for example, in New Mexico, 24 percent of births are midwife-attended.

Multiple large-scale studies have demonstrated the effectiveness and safety of the care midwives provide. In fact, American states with higher rates of midwifery integration have better birth outcomes. Freestanding birth centers with care provided by midwives increase positive outcomes for families as well. In 2014, the prestigious medical journal *The Lancet* released a landmark series highlighting midwifery and the power of midwives to improve outcomes.

MIDWIVES IN THE MEDIA

Birth is a spectacular event that can lend itself to lots of drama, so it's not surprising that it's frequently featured in films and TV shows—and often depicted in an exaggerated, negative way. Birth scenes often portray women writhing in agony and yelling at their loved ones. This can sneak its way into our collective understanding of birth, leading to fear that can hinder the experience for many people.

However, I would rather focus on positive and realistic representations of birth. One such example is *Call the Midwife: A Memoir of Birth, Joy, and Hard Times* by Jennifer Worth. This beautiful book and its two sequels have also been adapted into the wildly successful BBC show *Call the Midwife,* available in the United States on Netflix and PBS. This series is based on the true experiences of midwives from England in the 1950s. The stories shared on the show are powerful in their honesty, never presented as either overly glossy and saccharine or gloomy and fear-filled. Quite simply, the births represented are real: glorious and messy, mundane yet transformational. The series also highlights the exhausting and exhilarating work that midwives do every day to serve families.

What Does a Midwife Do?

A midwife is a practitioner whose expertise is in women's health and reproductive cycles. In particular, midwives are experts in what is "normal," meaning the natural physiologic process. Midwives view the process of pregnancy, labor, and birth as natural and healthy. They also offer care for healthy newborns and assistance with lactation. They provide independent care, meaning they're the primary medical provider throughout pregnancy; there won't be a physician present at prenatal appointments, at birth, in the immediate postpartum period, or through the first six weeks after a baby is born, unless special circumstances require it. Many midwives also offer full-scope, comprehensive care throughout the life cycle: annual check-ups (gynecological or otherwise), contraception, STI screening and prevention, breast exams, cancer screening, and menopause support. Depending on training, a midwife might even be able to prescribe medications to treat common obstetrical and gynecological issues.

WHAT QUALIFICATIONS DOES A MIDWIFE HAVE?

Choosing a midwife is a very individualized process. There are a few different types of midwife, each with slightly different certifications and education, but the letters after their name may matter less than their experience, practice style, and integration in the community. There are fantastic midwives in all credential types. This is why meeting midwives and finding one with whom you feel comfortable building a relationship is critical.

Certified nurse midwives (CNMs) have bachelor's degrees in general nursing and master's degrees in midwifery. CNMs are nationally certified through an organization called the American Midwifery Certification Board (AMCB), can legally practice in all states, and may have authority to write prescriptions for medications. CNMs may practice in hospitals, freestanding birth centers, and homes. With a wide scope of practice, they can offer care to some moderate- or higher-risk pregnancies as well as comprehensive health care outside pregnancy, including treatment of minor primary-care issues.

Certified midwives (CMs) do not have nursing degrees but have obtained a bachelor's degree in a related field and received intensive training in midwifery through a graduate program. Upon completion of their training, they take the same national exam through the AMCB that CNMs take. However, they are legally allowed to practice in only six states: New York, New Jersey, Rhode Island, Delaware, Maine, and Missouri.

Certified professional midwives (CPMs) have trained through various non-nursing paths. Typically, they follow a more direct apprenticeship model, working with an established midwife, but there are schools that offer a structured route to this certification as well. They must pass a national certification exam managed by the North American Registry for Midwives, but their credential is not legally recognized in every state. CPMs primarily focus on low-risk pregnancies and births that take place in birth centers and in the home.

Traditional and/or indigenous midwives train through their unique cultures and communities. They have a wealth of learned knowledge and specific insight into these communities and can often best recognize their needs. They may or may not be legally recognized to practice.

WHAT MAKES A MIDWIFE UNIQUE?

It's easy to be confused about the difference between doulas, midwives, and obstetricians, since they all share some overlap.

Midwifery and obstetrics both involve caring for pregnant people, but they're two very different professions with their own histories, philosophies, and training models. One is not better or worse than the other; they're simply distinct. Obstetricians are experts in pathology, or "abnormal" issues, such as pregnancies complicated by serious preexisting health conditions. They're also highly skilled surgeons who perform cesarean sections and other surgical procedures related to the female reproductive system. Midwives and obstetricians may work together in collaborative ways that can highlight the strengths and tools each provider type brings to the table.

Midwives and doulas, on the other hand, are both trained to support people through the process of pregnancy, labor, birth, and the postpartum period, providing emotional, psychological, and hands-on assistance. Unlike midwives, however, doulas do not have training as health care providers and cannot manage the clinical safety of their clients. This does not diminish the importance of doulas, as they can be a strong force for culturally competent care and in many cases can provide more direct one-on-one care than either a midwife or an obstetrician.

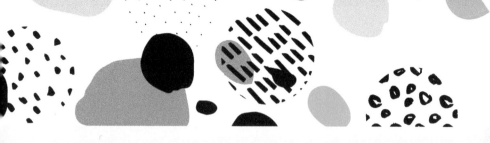

Birth Story: I CAN DO ANYTHING NOW

Miranda, who was having her first baby, had come to the birth center simply because we were in her neighborhood and accepted the state Medicaid insurance she had. At first, she and her family seemed unsure of our "weird" midwife ways. It was our responsibility to earn their trust and respect, and through time, dedication, and patience, we did.

When they arrived on the day of the birth, we had prepared the room with soft lights, aromatherapy, and a birth pool filled with nice warm water. Once inside, Miranda visibly relaxed and began to take full, deep breaths. Within minutes, she eased herself down into the pool and sighed in satisfaction.

Surrounded by her partner and family, Miranda was working hard but felt comfortable enough to let the process happen freely. Within two hours, she began the work of pushing and soon had progressed to crowning. Suddenly, she looked up at me and said, "I want to catch the baby myself." With the next contraction, Miranda confidently birthed her son into her hands. The room erupted into laughter, tears of joy, and hugs. Miranda glowed as love and pride radiated through her eyes and smile. Before leaving the center, she emphatically stated, "I can do anything now!"

Several months later, we had a new-pregnancy visit with Miranda's sister, who was now having her first baby. She'd been referred to us by Miranda's family, who had gone from being suspicious of our model to being full-fledged supporters!

The Benefits of Midwifery

Throughout this book, you'll encounter the term "care model" or "model of care." Simply defined, it means a specific system and set of principles used by health care professionals in caring for individuals. Different health care professions have different models of care.

In the midwifery model of care, families are respected as individuals and are given attention and care before pregnancy, throughout the childbearing year, and beyond. Midwives view health through a holistic lens and provide individualized care, honoring the dignity of each pregnant person while also monitoring for signs of potential complications. (If a serious complication arises, your midwife will consult with a physician.)

Choosing a midwife for care can be a wise approach in order to combine benefits from both the art and the science of women's health care. Here are a few of the many benefits of midwifery.

Midwifery is evidence-based. Midwifery is an ancient practice with deep roots, but that doesn't mean it's a relic of the past. It has always adapted and evolved to incorporate new knowledge, and modern midwifery combines the art and philosophy of women's health care with a strong understanding of science based in data and research. Midwifery can be a powerful way to achieve harmony between analyzing evidence-based medical information and applying it respectfully to the people we care for.

Midwifery care provides better health outcomes while being more cost-effective. According to Harvard's Maternal Health Task Force, the United States currently spends the most money per capita of any country in the world on providing maternity care—yet, sadly, still has the worst health outcomes of any developed nation. Midwifery care has consistently been proven to decrease rates of cesarean births, preterm births, significant perineal trauma, and low-birthweight babies while also increasing rates of breastfeeding and reducing the cost of care. It is often more cost-effective for individual families while also saving money for the health care system through improved outcomes.

People report higher levels of satisfaction with midwifery care. As providers, midwives believe that pregnant people and their families are capable of making the best choices for their own lives and care. We foster empowerment and autonomy through a practice called "informed consent and choice." This means that midwives are dedicated to educating families one-on-one about the procedures, tests, and processes they'll go through and fully addressing their questions and concerns. The solid, trusting relationship we build with families not only leads to a more robust and compassionate care model but also makes midwifery safer. Midwives have fewer preterm births, admissions to the NICU, low-birthweight babies, cesarean births, and instrumental/operative births (births using forceps and/or vacuum extraction) than obstetricians. This is because they truly know their clients throughout all the stages of pregnancy and birth. Due to the attention and respect they receive, midwifery clients report higher satisfaction rates and positive feelings about their birth experiences.

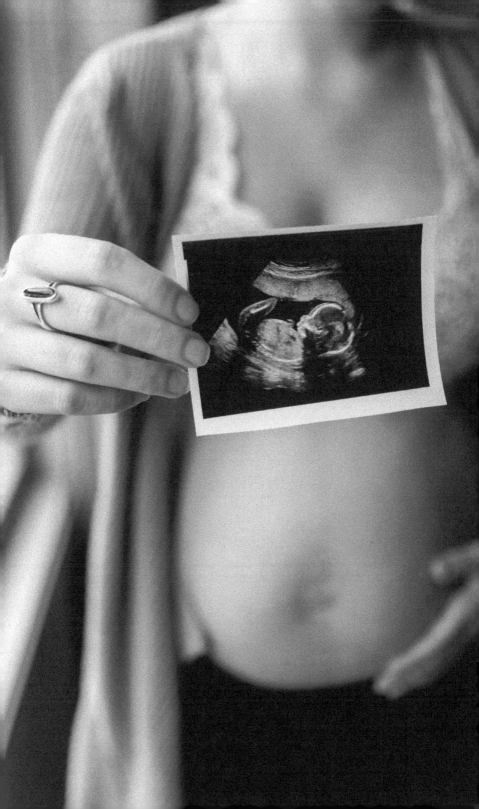

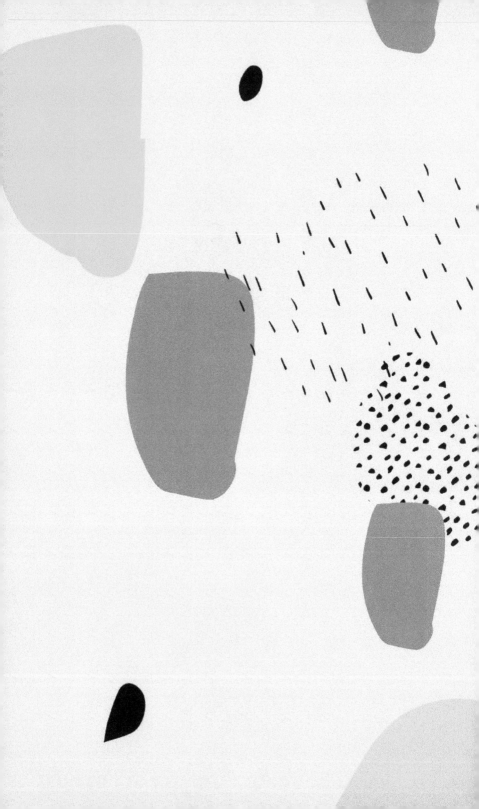

CHAPTER 2

Is Midwifery Right for Me?

As you begin your journey of pregnancy and parenting, you are the key decision maker. It is you who has the right to determine where and with whom you'll give birth—in a hospital, at home, or at a birth center, with a midwife or with a physician. The choice should and does belong to you and your family. In this chapter, we'll explore various options and decisions related to planning your pregnancy, labor, and birth, which can ultimately help you determine where you want to give birth, what kind of labor you want to plan on, and what kind of provider you want to work with.

Is Natural Childbirth Right for Me?

People often refer to unmedicated vaginal birth as "natural," but that term can have many different definitions and connotations attached to it. After all, it's not like a medicated birth is 100 percent "unnatural"—and "natural" isn't always necessarily better. For these reasons, I prefer the term "physiologic birth," which means trusting your body to go through labor and birth on its own power. It also refers to births that are not augmented or induced with pharmaceutical medications, for pain control or otherwise.

Why might you want a physiologic birth? In short, it allows and encourages your body to work in its most optimal way. Our bodies have been fine-tuned through the millennia to give birth, and if the process didn't work well overall, we wouldn't have billions of people on the planet. If you're healthy and your pregnancy has a low risk of complications— which, on average, most do—then the birthing process works best when we don't intervene.

Often, our interventions cause other issues to arise, which then require more interventions, and so on. This is referred to as the "cascade of interventions" and is a well-documented phenomenon in maternity care. For example, epidurals often cause a precipitous drop in blood pressure, which can affect the baby's heart rate and require additional medication to bring the blood pressure back up. While this drop is short-lived most of the time, sometimes the issue cannot be fixed and may require a surgical birth.

Having a physiologic birth does not mean that you simply suffer through pain or that you need superhuman pain tolerance. With proper support, education, and planning, this kind of birth is a very attainable goal. And with that planning and support, you will gain tools to help cope with the sensations of labor so that you don't suffer.

That said, not everyone will have a low-risk pregnancy, and not everyone will want a physiologic birth. What makes a birth empowering or positive is not the type or location. Rather, it is making fully informed choices that best suit you and your family. It's important to be clear about your desires and make choices that support them. Let's take a look at the factors that will help you determine whether a physiologic birth is right for you.

RISK LEVEL

Pregnancy risk level doesn't have a specific medical definition, so determining whether a pregnancy is low-, medium-, or high-risk is a nuanced situation. In general, there are several conditions that make your pregnancy moderate- or high-risk, including preexisting conditions such as diabetes, epilepsy, high blood pressure, heart disease, blood-clotting disorders, and severe asthma. Your risk factor can also be raised by conditions that develop during pregnancy, such as being pregnant with twins or triplets; pregnancy-related diabetes, high blood pressure, or preeclampsia; issues with the placenta; or identified concerns with the baby. These situations mean that your pregnancy needs intensive monitoring and that you have a higher risk of complications.

If you have or develop any of these complications, you may need medical intervention, so the safest plan is to prepare for a hospital birth—but depending on the specific concern and availability in your area, you may still be able to have a midwife attend your birth. Certified nurse midwives (CNMs) often work in hospital settings in collaboration with physicians and can continue to manage your care if the risk is moderate. If the complication is very high-risk, your midwife may need to transfer your care completely to a physician. (If you're working with a doula, they'll be able to continue working with you regardless of where and with whom you give birth.)

If you're healthy before you conceive, it's likely you'll remain healthy throughout the pregnancy and birth. Midwifery care is potentially a great fit for low-risk pregnancies like this; if you remain healthy throughout your pregnancy, a physiologic birth is a viable option.

PAIN MANAGEMENT

Pain management is an important factor to consider when planning your birth. There is no right or wrong choice here; birth is not a contest, and it's hard work, no matter how it happens. It's critical to be honest about what you want and plan accordingly.

Pain Management for Non-Physiologic Births

For non-physiologic births, the most common form of pain management is the epidural. When you get an epidural, a pump delivers a continuous dose of powerful pain medications (opioids, narcotics, and anesthetics) through a tiny tube into the space around the spinal cord (but not directly into it). This induces numbness from the waist down without affecting your mental state, which reduces the pain of giving birth but also means you won't be able to get out of bed or go to the bathroom on your own. Because of this, you'll urinate through a catheter, a hollow tube that goes through the urethra into the bladder, which will either be inserted intermittently or be left in until you're ready to push.

Epidurals can decrease the laboring person's blood pressure, which can negatively affect the baby's heart rate and pattern. When this happens, it can usually be reversed by medication, but sometimes it can't. Using an epidural can also cause the baby to have a harder time breastfeeding. More serious complications are rare, but they do happen. You can assess all these risk and benefits with your midwife as you make the important decision about whether to plan an epidural.

Epidurals are administered by either a physician (an anesthesiologist) or an advanced-practice nurse (a certified registered nurse anesthetist) and are therefore only an option in hospital births—but that doesn't mean you can't use a midwife. Midwives who work in hospital settings can offer their clients epidurals and intravenous pain medication.

Pain Management for Physiologic Births

Physiologic births don't use pharmaceutical pain management, but that doesn't mean they don't incorporate any methods for reducing pain. Midwives might use techniques like water immersion and water birth, massage, positional changes, aromatherapy, and herbal mixtures that can soothe anxiety and promote relaxation. These options are more common in birth-center or home births but are sometimes available in hospitals as well.

Another option is nitrous oxide, also known as laughing gas. Though some would argue that the use of nitrous means the labor is no longer unmedicated or physiologic, I would say that it is still physiologic, as the nitrous doesn't interfere with the hormonal process of the body and the person using it is still in full control of their body and mind.

If you want a physiologic birth, I recommend choosing a provider and setting that support this option as well as enrolling in a comprehensive class on natural birth. In my experience, those who choose an unmedicated birth and prepare thoroughly are usually successful. Educate yourself well and be honest about what you truly want, and you can feel confident in your decision. It's all about identifying what is important to you and your family and then consciously choosing the options that best fit those desires.

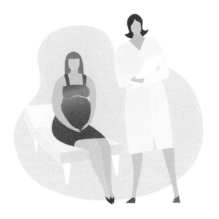

WATER IMMERSION AND WATER BIRTH

Water immersion, also called hydrotherapy, is when a person who is in labor sits in a birthing pool filled with warm water for comfort and relaxation—kind of like taking a nice soak in a hot tub. *Water birth* is when the birth itself occurs in the birthing pool. Both are great forms of physiologic pain management and result in improved coping during labor, improved maternal satisfaction, and decreased rates of first- and second-degree lacerations (tears in the vulvar, vaginal, or perineal area that occur during birth). At my birth center, about 90 percent of clients use hydrotherapy, and 40 percent have water births.

You might wonder: Doesn't delivering in water put the baby at risk of drowning? But there is little risk in water birth for a number of reasons. Newborns are actually stimulated to take their first breath by the feeling of air on their skin, so they don't inhale until lifted from the pool. Second, humans' natural "dive reflex" prevents us from inhaling when submerged in water. (This is why young babies can take swim classes and be briefly submerged without drowning.) Finally, when the baby first emerges, they are still receiving oxygen through the umbilical cord, so they don't need to breathe immediately. When managed by competent, well-trained providers, water birth is very safe for healthy, low-risk laboring people.

VAGINAL BIRTH

Giving birth vaginally is the most physiologic or "natural" way to have a baby. When a healthy pregnant person receives good prenatal care, a vaginal birth typically offers them easier recovery postpartum, as the body can heal quicker from a vaginal birth than from a surgical birth.

Vaginal birth is also very beneficial for the baby. The birth canal helps push the fluid out of babies' lungs so they can breathe air once they're born. It also exposes newborns to their mothers' bacteria and other microbes, which lays the foundation for a healthy gut and immune system.

CESAREAN SECTION BIRTH

A cesarean section, or C-section, is when a surgeon cuts open a pregnant person's abdomen to deliver the baby directly from the uterus rather than the baby being pushed out through the vagina. (It's named after Julius Caesar, who was supposedly delivered this way.) These surgeries can absolutely save lives, and it's crucial to have access to them in the event of certain complications, including significant fetal distress in labor, placental abruption (when the placenta comes off the uterine wall prior to birth), placenta previa (when the placenta has grown over the cervix), or severe medical complications with the birthing parent.

However, the United States has a national C-section rate of 32 percent, which is dramatically higher than what you'd expect given that C-sections are recommended in less than 15 percent of births. This is important to know because a C-section isn't risk-free; it's a major abdominal surgery. In the short term, there are risks for injury, infection, and bleeding. In the long term, having a C-section increases the risks of lowered fertility, pain with sexual intercourse, and severe complications with future pregnancies. There are also increased risks for babies delivered via C-section, such as asthma, allergies, obesity, and difficulty initiating breastfeeding. Because of these potential problems, C-sections should be reserved for the instances that truly warrant them.

One way to help ensure that you only get a C-section if you really need one is to receive care from a midwife. For example, in freestanding birth centers where care is supervised by midwives, the cesarean rate is much lower than average—approximately 4 to 6 percent of births require a C-section—while favorable outcomes for both women and babies are still maintained. If a C-section does become necessary, obstetricians are expert surgeons who can intervene and save lives. Midwives do not perform cesarean sections, though some hospital-based midwives have received additional training and can assist the physician as part of the surgical team.

MAKING DECISIONS TOGETHER

The most important member of your birth team, other than you, is your partner. This partner can be the other parent, a trusted family member, or even a doula. Whoever it is, it's important to have this support because regardless of how you decide to give birth, it's an intense transition that will benefit from a team approach. Afterward, you'll need help caring for both the baby and yourself. It truly does take a village. Identifying and gathering your village starts with your birth partner.

Your partner should be as involved as they can be. A good first step is for them to accompany you to as many of your prenatal appointments as possible. Partners should also attend any and all classes you take. I highly recommend a comprehensive childbirth-preparation class, a breastfeeding class, and a class on newborn care and safety. After birth and in the first few weeks postpartum, you may be exhausted and overwhelmed, so it's critical to have a support person who had all the same education as you. Together, you can remember the most important things you need to know.

Where Do I Want to Give Birth?

There are three main settings in which to give birth: at home, at a freestanding birth center, or at a hospital. Many families associate midwives only with home birth, but depending on their training, midwives can attend births in all settings. Currently, in the United States, over 90 percent of births happen in a hospital, while only up to 4 percent happen at home or at a birth center. Wherever you decide to have your baby, you should be able to have a midwife at your birth. Let's take a look at all three options to help you decide which one is right for you.

GIVING BIRTH AT HOME

If your pregnancy is low-risk and you have a trained midwife at your side, giving birth at home can be a very safe choice. Like every choice, it has pros and cons. One obvious big benefit to home birth is that it's your home—a place where you feel comfortable and are surrounded by familiar things. The midwife comes to you, so you don't need to travel in your car while you're in labor.

For some families, though, a home birth isn't ideal. Perhaps you live in an apartment and your landlord is against the idea, or maybe you don't feel like your home situation is safe. Another stumbling block may be how far away you live from a hospital; in the unlikely event that a transfer becomes necessary, it's a good idea to be within about 30 minutes of a hospital.

If you do choose a home birth, your midwife will do at least one home visit during your prenatal care to be sure she's familiar with your home and how to get there. She'll also give you a list of supplies to have ready for the birth (some common household items plus some that need to be specially ordered) but will bring the necessary medical equipment and supplies herself. Home-birth midwifery may not be covered by your insurance, and most families pay for the services themselves out of pocket.

GIVING BIRTH AT A BIRTH CENTER

For many families, choosing a birth center feels like a good middle ground between home and hospital. Birth centers have excellent outcomes for both mom and baby in low-risk pregnancies, and because they're run by midwives, they can truly follow the midwifery model of care.

Some advantages to birth centers include large, cozy birth pools, comfortable home-like surroundings, and alternative pain-management options that may not be available in a hospital or home setting, like nitrous oxide. Additionally, most birth centers have good relationships with local hospitals, are located relatively close to them, and have strong transfer protocols in place, all of which can save time and confusion in the rare event of an emergency.

One of the only downsides to choosing a birth center is that you have to drive there. Traveling in the car while you're in labor is not a fun experience. But the birth-center midwives will have clear instructions about the travel and ways to cope with the transition.

Note that while some birth centers may be fully covered by private insurance and Medicaid, others may not. This will be an important question to ask of each center as part of your decision-making process.

GIVING BIRTH AT A HOSPITAL
WITH A MIDWIFE

Giving birth in a hospital with a midwife can also be a good choice, particularly if you have conditions that make your pregnancy moderate-risk or if you think you may want an epidural. (Choosing an epidural does not mean that you can no longer work with a midwife; hospital-based midwives can offer this option.) Hospitals are frequently covered by private insurance and Medicaid, though you want to confirm that they take your specific plan. Additionally, larger urban or suburban hospitals are staffed by all-emergency personnel 24 hours a day.

There are also some potential drawbacks to planning a hospital birth. Hospitals are large institutions, so getting individualized care—care that incorporates your history and focuses on you as a whole person rather than as "the patient in room 27"—can be challenging. Much of the care is provided by the nursing staff, and you likely won't meet any of them ahead of time. At small community or rural hospitals, you may not have in-house emergency staff 24 hours a day. You'll also have to travel there when you're in labor, which, as stated previously, can be unpleasant but is definitely still doable.

How Do I Pay for Midwifery Care?

This is a common question, and with good reason. I've been working in this field for many years and can still find the situation confusing. Here are the answers to some of the questions that come up most often.

Will my private insurance cover a midwife? The answer depends on both the type of midwife and the type of insurance. If you plan to give birth in a hospital with a CNM, then the answer is likely yes. If you plan to give birth in your home or at a freestanding birth center, then it can vary widely. Some insurance plans cover certified professional midwives (CPMs), and some don't. Some birth centers work with insurance companies, and some don't. You'll need to clarify with your individual insurance and the specific provider you're considering.

Does state Medicaid insurance cover a midwife? This answer is very similar to the one for the previous question. If you're planning a hospital birth with a CNM, the answer is probably yes. Otherwise, it depends on the specific state, provider type, and planned location of birth.

What if I don't have insurance and will be paying out of pocket? In this case, the most cost-effective option will likely be working with a midwife who attends home births or works with a birth center. Having an uncomplicated vaginal birth in a US hospital costs $11,000 to $12,000 on average—and that doesn't include any of your prenatal or postpartum care. This is easily two to three times more expensive than the cost of comprehensive care—including prenatal care, labor, birth, and postpartum care—with a midwife at home or at a birth center.

There's one very important fact you should know in advance about birth and insurance billing in the United States: There are two separate items that insurance companies bill. The first is the *provider fee*, which is the cost for your provider (either a midwife or physician) to give you your full prenatal care, attend your birth, and provide your postpartum care. The second is the *facility fee*, which is the cost to use a facility—a birth center or hospital—for the birth itself. (Depending on the situation, a home birth might have a facility fee as well, which your insurance may or may not cover.) In general, the facility fee for a hospital birth is up to three or four times higher than the facility fee for a birth center. In this case, if you have a high-deductible plan, choosing a birth center may be more cost-effective for your family.

I know this may leave you with more questions than answers, and I am sorry for that. Unfortunately, in our current health care system, figuring out costs and insurance can be a convoluted situation. It's important for you as the consumer to advocate for yourself and demand clarity from both your insurance company and your provider. Remember that you are the consumer and that each entity owes you a straightforward and transparent explanation of the billing process.

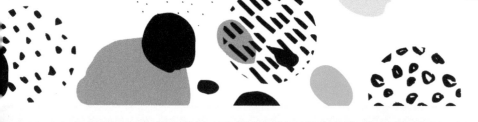

Birth Story: IN COMPLETE CONTROL

It was Amber's second birth. The first had been with me at
another birth center. During that labor, she had used nitrous
oxide (laughing gas) to help with pain management, and it had
been extremely beneficial for her. One of her main concerns
with this second birth was to have the option of nitrous oxide
again, so when she called in labor, I was sure to get the equipment set up and ready.

Amber and her partner, Luis, arrived at the birth center. She
was in good, active labor with strong, regular contractions. All
laboring people have a power that radiates through them, and
some also have a glow. Amber had the glow. Luis was wonderful, present and attentive. Amber's fantastic doula, Jennifer,
brought a calm strength to the process. The room was full of so
much love and support. Amber wanted hands-on contact and
closeness, and I was struck multiple times by the vision of us
all circling around her, lifting up her spirit and adding strength
to her process.

As she neared transition—the time just before pushing
begins, when the intensity really kicks up—she asked for
nitrous oxide. For her, it offered a calmness and ability to focus
on the work. She used it perfectly, breathing it in during her
contractions and taking a break from it in between contractions. Amber spent time in the birth pool, on the bed, and on
the birth stool, all the while using the nitrous oxide to help her
relax and let the contractions do their task. One of the great
things about nitrous oxide is that the laboring person is in

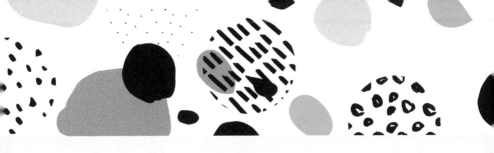

complete control of it: how much to use, when to use it, and when to stop.

Then she started pushing, working to bring her baby earthside. She was full of power and channeled it through her efforts, saying, "My body can do this!" as a mantra. Soon, her healthy, vigorous baby was welcomed to the world and placed skin to skin on her chest.

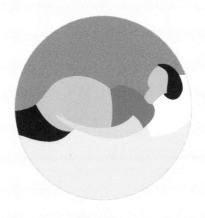

Finding a Midwife

So you're thinking a midwife sounds right for you—but how do you go about finding one? There are many ways to connect with the right midwife. Keep in mind that where you decide to give birth will have a bearing on what type of midwife you hire; CNMs and CMs can work in homes, birth centers, and hospitals, while CPMs usually work in homes and birth centers but not in hospitals.

WHERE TO START

A great way to start looking for a midwife is by asking people in your community who have had midwifery care. Local parenting, lactation, and pregnancy groups—either in person or through social media—can also be great reference sources. If you're working with private insurance, you can consult your plan for a list of approved midwives.

Most states have associations for midwives, which can be found by searching "[your state] midwife association" online. You can also connect with local midwives through national organizations' websites. The American College of Nurse Midwives (ACNM) has a "Find a Midwife" tab on their website, and there's a similar "Find a Birth Center" tab on the website of the American Association of Birth Centers (AABC). Finally, a good old-fashioned Google search of "midwife in my area" can be effective as well.

WHEN TO START

Some families work with a midwife before they even conceive, by going through preconception counseling. Preconception counseling involves a face-to-face visit and exam to evaluate your overall health status and screen for potential issues. Other families start care with a midwife as soon as they have a positive home pregnancy test. And others, perhaps unhappy with the care they're receiving from a physician, begin working with a midwife weeks or months into their pregnancy. There's no right or wrong time to start midwifery care, but in general, the sooner the better—this will give you the time to develop a good relationship with your midwife. It's also ideal to start prenatal care early in the first trimester, regardless of who's providing that care. Midwives offer the same testing and screening as obstetricians, so it's not necessary to see one before seeing a midwife. (If you have a low-risk pregnancy, you can go through your whole pregnancy seeing only a midwife and never working with a physician!)

WHAT TO LOOK FOR

Pregnancy, labor, birth, and postpartum are times of great importance and vulnerability, so your midwife should be someone you feel comfortable with. An interview can be critical in determining who's a good fit for you. Most private midwives offer a free consultation visit where you can sit with them and ask questions, and freestanding birth centers offer orientations or meet-and-greet sessions, usually led by a midwife, that are free and open to the public. These are also opportunities to tour the center and ask questions.

Humans all come with our own personalities, styles, and quirks, and midwives are no different. You'll want to find one who feels right to you. For example, if your religion is important to you, you may want to find a midwife who shares the same beliefs. If you're a person of color, it may be important to you that your midwife is also a person of color. Here are some sample questions you might ask a prospective midwife (it can be helpful to write them down ahead of time):

- *How many births have you attended?* This is not necessarily all about the number—you mainly just want to make sure that they're up-front and comfortable with their level of experience.

- *Where did you receive your training, and how long have you been in practice?* Again, any provider should be open and honest about their training.

- *What are your protocols for responding to an emergency? What emergency equipment and medications will you have available?* This is particularly important for midwives who work in the community setting (at homes or birth centers). The midwife should have relationships with local emergency medical services and hospitals. They should also be able to detail the medications and equipment they have for first-line measures for both mother and baby.

- *How often do you end up transferring clients to the hospital?* In my personal practice as a birth-center midwife, my transfer rate in labor is around 11 percent, which is in line with national birth-center statistics and international guidelines. In a population of low-risk people who start spontaneous labor, around 10 to 15 percent of them will go on to require a higher level of care, so the transfer rate for community births should ideally be within that range.

- *What is your cesarean birth rate?* Of course, midwives do not perform cesarean sections, but what percentage of their clients have needed one?

- *What is your rate of perineal lacerations, and do you feel comfortable suturing those lacerations?* Perineal lacerations are tears that can happen in the labia, vagina, and/or perineum during the birth process.

- *Who do you collaborate with?* Every midwife should have a strong network of providers they can consult and collaborate with. These should include obstetricians as well as pediatricians if the midwife provides newborn care.

- *What plans do you have in place if you have two clients in labor at the same time?* A home-birth midwife should have other midwives they can call in to assist in these situations, while a birth center should have plans to cover multiple births by having more midwives available as needed. If this is a midwife who works in a hospital, are there other midwives who will back them up, or will physicians do that?

RED FLAGS

Finding a midwife who "feels" right is important. It's also important to choose a midwife who is well rooted in the local community and practices in a manner that fosters safety. When looking at prospective midwives, ask yourself: What is their reputation in the community? Do they share reviews or testimonials on their website? Are they integrated in the local health system? Do they have a strong network of other providers to consult with? Are they approachable and open about their practice, or do they become defensive when asked questions? Are they involved in continuing education and their local and national professional organizations? What do they do to make sure they're current with the latest data?

A big red flag is a midwife who thinks they don't need a strong network. A midwife who is a "lone wolf" may be one for a reason, and that reason could be that they practice outside the realm of established and recognized care models. Credentials alone do not guarantee a reliable, conscientious provider. All types of providers—physicians and midwives alike—can potentially provide care that is not up-to-date with evidence-based guidelines. Consumers should never choose a provider based solely on the letters after their name.

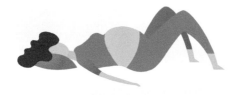

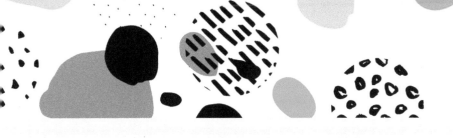

Birth Story: DANCE PARTY

Stacie was having her second baby and her first at our birth center. Her partner, Tri, and her doula, Emily, were present and supportive. Stacie's labor was strong, with frequent, powerful contractions, but the process was taking longer than expected because the baby was in a position known as a "posterior presentation," which means that the baby's face is looking at the mother's pubic bone instead of her back. Babies in this position can still be delivered through physiologic birth, but it can make labor longer and cause more discomfort.

I wanted to try some interventions to turn the baby over—something I knew an actively laboring woman wouldn't be thrilled to hear. I discussed the plan with Emily, and then we went over it with Stacie and her husband. Stacie wasn't too excited, but she wanted to have her baby, so she agreed. Over the next hour, we had Stacie get on her hands and knees, rock on a birth ball, do side lunges with one leg up on a step stool, and walk up and down stairs. All the while, Emily and Tri were there to offer Stacie support and encouragement. At one point, when Stacie was really frustrated, Emily pulled out her phone and played one of Stacie's favorite songs, and we all had an impromptu dance party. It was exactly what we needed to change up the heavy energy. Soon after, the baby made a big turn, and Stacie felt the urge to push. We moved back to the birth room and prepared. Shortly afterward, her gorgeous baby was born into her partner's waiting hands, welcomed with love and joy.

Do I Want a Doula?

No matter where you choose to give birth or who your provider is, a doula can be a valuable part of your team. Doulas are not trained health care providers and are not responsible for overseeing your physical health and safety, so they can't take the place of either a midwife or a physician. But their support can be a great addition to your birth experience.

WHAT DOES A DOULA DO?

A doula is a trained professional who specializes in providing emotional, psychological, and educational support to pregnant women and postpartum families. Doulas also provide hands-on physical support during your birth, including positional suggestions (to help alleviate discomfort or put the baby into a favorable position) and comfort measures (such as massage). Many doulas also have additional training in lactation and newborn care—in fact, there are doulas who specialize in postpartum care and support in addition to or instead of pregnancy and labor support. Doulas may provide in-home, nonmedical prenatal visits to help you develop a birth plan; offer private natural-birth education; and give suggestions on how to find evidence-based guidelines for many issues.

Doulas can work side by side with your provider, and their work can be integrated into your birth plans. Regardless of your planned place of birth or if those plans have to be altered, a doula remains with you and your family. If you plan a home birth with a midwife but develop a complication that requires you to transfer care to a physician at a hospital, a doula can make that change with you. If you start your pregnancy with a high-risk condition that will require a hospital birth with a physician, a doula can help maintain the personal care and touches that promote well-being during a stressful time. If you'll get your midwifery care through a hospital-based group, the midwife may not be able to be present with you for your entire labor process; in that case, a doula can give you and your family the comfort of having someone who's always present.

Many partners are concerned that a doula will take their place or make them feel unneeded. This could not be further from the truth. A good doula will facilitate your partner's support of you, educating and guiding them through the process. A doula works for both you and your partner and makes sure your partner is also well cared for.

HOW DO I FIND A DOULA?

As with finding a midwife, there are various ways to locate a doula, including asking for recommendations from friends and family or searching for doulas in your area online. Many regions also have local doula organizations that can offer referrals. Once you've chosen a provider, they can also be a valuable resource for doula services in your area. Midwives in particular are often aware of the doulas in the area and may have personal experience with them. Some providers only work with certain doulas who they know and have a relationship with, so be sure to ask if this is the case for your provider.

Working with a doula is an intimate experience, so it's crucial to find someone with whom you and your partner feel comfortable. Doulas usually offer a free consultation visit so you and your partner have a chance to meet them and ask questions.

Some doulas are trained through national certification organizations, while others are not. There is no national regulation of doula services, and the pros and cons of formal certification are different for each doula. When you're interviewing a potential doula, they should be comfortable talking about why they did or did not become certified. You should also understand their background and be comfortable with their training. It's important to hire a doula with whom both you and your partner feel comfortable, so take your time and plan to interview more than one.

Personality traits matter, and if you or your partner don't click with a doula, no matter the reason, then they likely won't be a good choice for you. Interview more than one doula so you can compare pricing and styles. Some doulas only work with clients who are planning a home or birth-center birth, while others may only work with clients who are planning a hospital birth; this will be an important topic to discuss when conducting an interview.

It's also important to remember that although some states are beginning to mandate coverage, most insurance companies don't cover any part of the cost of doula services. The price largely depends on the area where you live, but you'll likely pay between $300 and $1,500.

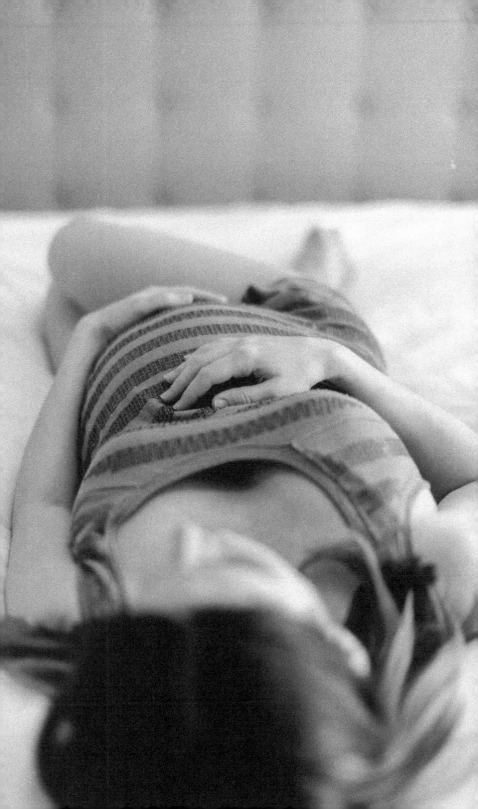

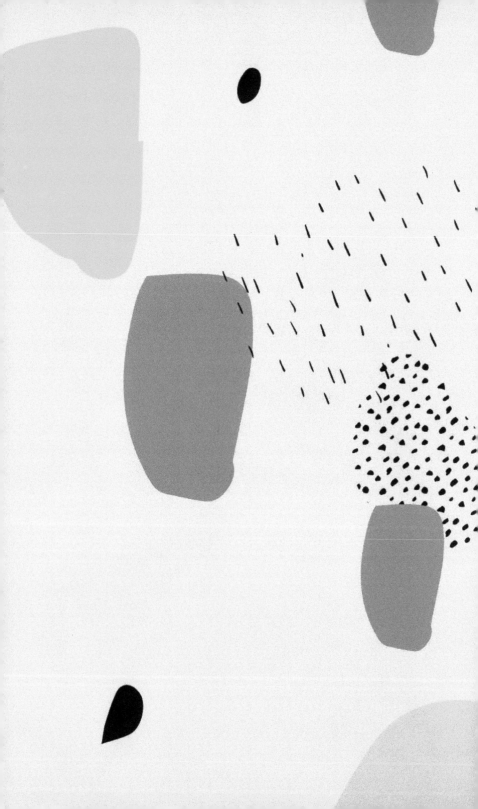

CHAPTER 3

Midwifery While You're Pregnant

Of course, midwives are best known for the work they do during labor and birth. However, their work starts well before that and continues after the baby is delivered. Midwives work with women and families from preconception through the 40 weeks of pregnancy and beyond. This chapter will focus on how your midwife will help guide, educate, and empower you through your pregnancy, monitoring the progress of your journey and, if necessary, intervening to ensure your health and safety.

A Pregnancy Primer

Conception and pregnancy are two of the most complex natural processes that we as humans accomplish. The fact that they happen every second of every day, all over the world, only serves to highlight how amazing our bodies are. Unfortunately, our current mainstream culture bombards us with negative messages about female bodies and misinformation about how they work. Let's take a brief look at how our bodies work and what does (and doesn't) happen during pregnancy.

YOUR BODY

Let's start with a simple overview of the basic structures that make up the female reproductive system, from the outside in.

The external genitalia are made up of the clitoris, labia majora (the thicker outer lips), and labia minora (the thinner inner lips). The labia help cover the opening of the vagina as well as the urethra (the opening where urine is released when you pee). The external genitalia are referred to singularly as the vulva. The perineum is the space between the vulva and the anus.

The external vaginal opening is located behind the labia, below the urethra. The vagina is the canal that leads from the vulva to the uterus (or "womb"), but it's not just an open tube. Rather, it's what is referred to as a "potential space," meaning that it closes in on itself when it's at rest. The tissue of the vagina is both strong and flexible, able to grow and shrink to meet the various needs it fulfills—for example, accommodating a penis during sexual intercourse, expelling menstrual blood (and fitting menstrual cups or tampons) during your period, and, of course, giving birth to a baby.

Internally, at the top of the vagina, is the cervix. The cervix is the gateway to the uterus, containing a canal that opens to the vagina on one side and the uterus on the other. Made of collagen and smooth muscle, it's one of the most adaptable parts of the human body. Semen enters the uterus through the cervix, and menstrual blood leaves the uterus through it as well. The strength of the cervix is also what keeps the baby, placenta, and all the uterine contents in the womb throughout the pregnancy. Because it is so strong, once labor begins, the cervix takes a while to soften and open enough to allow the baby to pass through—anywhere from a few hours to a few days.

Above the vagina, on the other side of the cervix, is the uterus. The uterus is roughly the size and shape of an

FEMALE REPRODUCTIVE SYSTEM

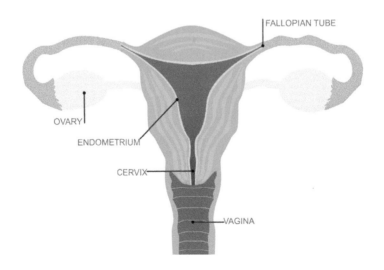

FALLOPIAN TUBE

OVARY

ENDOMETRIUM

CERVIX

VAGINA

upside-down pear. It is made of multiple layers of smooth muscle that overlap and wrap around the uterine cavity (which, unlike the vagina, is not a potential space and does stay open). During the menstrual cycle, the uterine lining, or endometrium, builds up a layer of temporary, nutrient-rich tissue. If a pregnancy happens, this lining helps form the placenta, which nourishes the fertilized egg as it grows into an embryo and then a fetus. If a pregnancy doesn't happen, the lining is shed through the cervix and out of the vagina as menstrual blood.

At the top of the uterus are two ovaries, one on either side, connected to the uterus by tubes called fallopian tubes. Roughly the size of almonds, the ovaries are the home to a woman's ova, or eggs. (Amazingly, all the eggs a woman will ever make are produced when she's still inside her own mother's womb and are already present in her ovaries by the time she's born.) Starting during puberty, the ovaries release approximately one egg per month. This egg travels into the fallopian tube, where it may encounter sperm and become fertilized. If it's not fertilized, it's expelled along with the uterine lining during a menstrual period. If it is fertilized, it completes the journey down into the uterus, where it will implant and grow over the next 40 weeks.

YOUR BABY

The growth and development of your baby is fascinating and complicated. A full-term pregnancy can last anywhere from 37 to 42 weeks. Your estimated due date falls at 40 weeks, but that's only an estimate; your baby can safely arrive anytime in that period.

Pregnancies are broken down into three periods of time, known as trimesters, and each trimester is filled with unique milestones for both the developing baby and the pregnant person.

The First Trimester: Conception to Week 12

The first trimester is one of rapid growth and development. The egg is fertilized in the fallopian tube, at which point it is no longer an egg but a zygote: a new, unique cell created by the fusion of the ovum and the sperm. As it travels down the tube and into the uterine cavity, it becomes a blastocyst (a zygote that has developed slightly). About 10 to 11 days after fertilization, the blastocyst implants into the uterine wall and becomes an embryo.

The first eight weeks after fertilization, known as the "embryonic period," are crucial, as this is when all the embryo's internal and external structures, from limbs to internal organs, are developed. The embryo develops from the head down—so, for example, the arms develop approximately one week before the legs. By six weeks after your last menstrual period, the cluster of cells that will become the heart starts to beat and can be seen by ultrasound. At the ninth week, the conclusion of the embryonic period, the embryo is now called a fetus, and the rest of the pregnancy is known as the "fetal period."

During the first trimester, all babies develop at a well-defined rate and pattern of growth, hitting certain developmental landmarks in a specific order. Between weeks 7 and 10 is a great time to use ultrasound to help view those developments and determine or verify your due date. After this period of time, growth won't be so uniform, as it will be influenced by the baby's unique genetics. For instance, petite parents might produce a short, petite person, while lankier parents might produce a taller, lankier child. Because of that, the further along you are in your pregnancy, the less useful an ultrasound is at accurately determining a due date.

The Second Trimester: Week 13 to Week 26

The second trimester is also a time of growth. Cartilage turns into bone as the baby's skeleton begins to form. The baby also starts to grow in size, which causes the uterus to stretch and become thinner. Due to this growth and thinned-out uterus, pregnant people experience a phenomenon known as "quickening." This is the first experience of feeling the baby move and usually happens around 18 to 20 weeks after your last menstrual period.

The second trimester is also the time when you can use an ultrasound to find out the fetus's sex. Many providers, midwives included, offer to do a specific ultrasound called an anatomy scan, which lets you see the baby's external and internal systems and check them for possible concerns. At the end of this trimester, the average baby will weigh 1.25 pounds.

The Third Trimester: Week 27 to Birth

The third trimester is the trimester of finishing touches. Babies start to grow hair, have rhythmic breathing movements, respond to light and sound, and control their movements. They may even suck their thumbs! Lungs fully develop as the baby prepares to begin breathing air. The brain undergoes significant growth, tripling in weight over this trimester. By the end of this period, the average baby weighs 7 pounds and 5 ounces.

1 MONTH

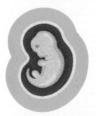

2 MONTHS

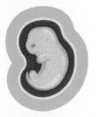

3 MONTHS

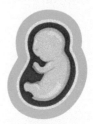

4 MONTHS

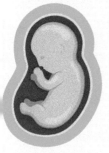

5 MONTHS

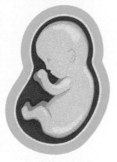

6 MONTHS

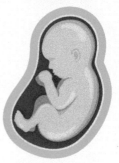

7 MONTHS

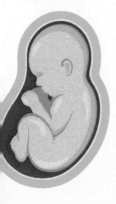

8 MONTHS

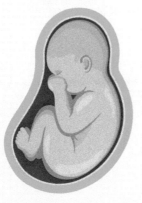

9 MONTHS

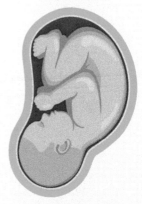

The Role of the Midwife during Pregnancy

During pregnancy, your midwife will oversee many things, monitoring your health as well as the health of your baby. A midwife offers all the same testing and screening that a doctor would, including blood tests and ultrasounds. But you'll also notice some distinct differences from physician-based care. Midwives focus on one-on-one education with families and typically spend more face-to-face time with their clients in order to explain development and answer questions. They also usually offer diet and exercise counseling and have a strong focus on the mental health of their clients.

Most pregnant people who choose care with a midwife won't need to see a physician during the pregnancy. If your midwife has concerns or you develop a complication, then they'll consult with a physician. All midwives should have physicians whom they can consult with and refer clients to when needed. Depending on the individual midwife, their practice setting, and the specific concern or complication, your midwife may be able to co-manage your care, or they may need to transfer your care completely to a physician.

Prenatal Checkups with a Midwife

Getting regular prenatal care is essential to a healthy pregnancy. It's generally recommended to start seeing your provider early in your pregnancy, around 8 to 10 weeks after your last menstrual period. This first visit is very important to both establish your medical care and begin building a relationship with your provider. If you've opted to receive care from a midwife at this point, it won't be necessary to also see a physician or other provider. If you started care with another provider and now want to transfer to a midwife, the midwife won't need to repeat any of the previous care, but you will have to fill out a special form to request your records from your previous provider.

Depending on the type of midwife you're seeing, prenatal visits may take place in your home or in the midwife's office. If you're planning a birth-center birth, the appointments will likely take place at the center, while if you're planning a hospital birth, your appointments will likely happen at a more "typical"-looking medical office.

THE FIRST VISIT

This first visit will cover a lot of ground, which is why it's usually much longer than subsequent visits. A typical first visit might include the following:

Medical history. Your midwife will take a comprehensive look at your personal medical history and the medical histories of close relatives, including your siblings and parents.

Physical exam. Your midwife will listen to your heart and lungs; check your reflexes; feel your abdomen, thyroid, and lymph nodes; and otherwise assess your physical health.

Breast and/or pelvic exam. Depending on your personal history and needs, the midwife may offer to do a clinical breast exam or a pelvic exam and Pap smear. These more invasive procedures should be thoroughly discussed and only performed with your consent.

Reproductive history. Your midwife will ask about your menstrual cycle and any previous pregnancies and then use that information to establish an initial estimated due date (EDD).

Blood draw. You'll likely have your blood drawn for lab tests that screen for anemia, blood-borne diseases, and immunity to communicable diseases. These tests will also determine your blood type.

Ultrasound. Depending on your history, you may be offered an ultrasound to help verify your EDD. This ultrasound can be very helpful if you're unsure of the date of your last period or if you have irregular cycles.

Genetic testing. Another important component of this first visit is a discussion pertaining to genetic screening and testing. Some of this testing will look directly at the baby, while some will look at your risks. Whether or not to pursue genetic screening is a big and very personal decision and one that should be made with care after thorough explanation from your midwife. The ultimate choice is yours; some families opt to do all the testing as soon as possible, while other families choose to do no testing at all. There is no "right" answer.

MONTHLY CHECKUPS

Following the first appointment with your midwife, you'll see them approximately once per month for the next few months. These appointments will involve more counseling, education, and discussion of your baby's development as well as the progression of your pregnancy. The midwife will assess your blood pressure, listen to the baby's heartbeat, and check in about what you're eating and how much exercise you're getting. They'll ask about how you're feeling, both physically and emotionally, and will offer anticipatory guidance on what to expect in the coming weeks between visits. They'll also go over the results of any testing from that first visit and, if necessary, recommend interventions or support based on those results. Midwives are experts in the most common discomforts of each stage of pregnancy, so they'll help guide you through those as well.

THIRD-TRIMESTER VISITS

At the start of your third trimester, you'll begin to have more frequent visits with your midwife—typically at 28, 30, 32, 34, and 36 weeks and then once a week until you give birth. At around 28 weeks, you'll probably receive some recommended screenings for anemia and a condition called gestational diabetes, both of which are assessed through bloodwork. At each visit, your midwife will continue to monitor your blood pressure, assess fetal health, and listen to the baby's heartbeat. As you progress in your pregnancy, visits will begin to cover labor and birth concerns. You'll plan and review your preferences and goals with your midwife and get suggestions on coping with common end-of-pregnancy discomforts. You'll also be educated on potential dangers and symptoms that you should immediately alert your midwife to, including rashes, unusual headaches, and decreased fetal movement.

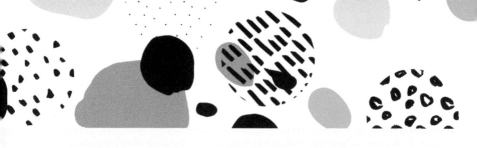

Birth Story: THE FEAST

After a year of trying to conceive, Morgan and her partner, Dan, were ecstatic to finally have that positive home pregnancy test. But seven or eight weeks into her pregnancy, Morgan began to experience nausea and vomiting. At first, she was able to manage it with traditional home remedies such as sour hard candies, acupressure wrist bands, and eating small, protein-focused meals and snacks throughout the day. But as the pregnancy progressed, Morgan's nausea became significantly worse. She began to have such a hard time keeping down food and fluids that she started to lose weight. Her "routine" morning sickness had progressed to a more severe condition: hyperemesis gravidarum.

We prescribed her a strong medication to help control the vomiting, and she made frequent trips to the hospital for intravenous fluids and nutrients. She had a supportive birth team, but she still struggled to get through each day.

Her labor started at 38 weeks, and, amazingly, once the contractions started, the constant nausea and vomiting just melted away. For her, labor was a massive relief. It was beautiful to watch the light come back into her eyes! Dan was brought to tears many times throughout the process as he watched his partner return to herself. Just over seven hours after her first contraction, she and Dan welcomed their gorgeous baby to the world.

Then Morgan began to have the biggest post-birth feast I have ever seen. She not only enjoyed the post-birth meal

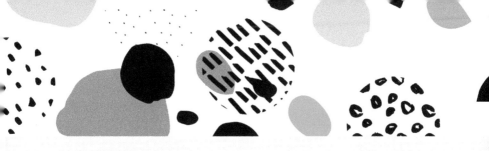

we make for our families at the birth center, she also had her family and friends go pick up more food. The birth room was full of almost every type of food you can imagine. Morgan, glowing, with her baby curled up skin to skin on her chest, was satisfied on every level.

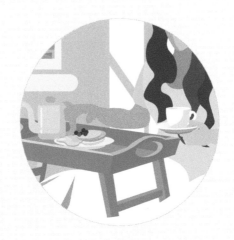

Pregnancy with a Doula

Incorporating a doula into your care team as a nonmedical support provider can be a valuable decision. Families usually bring a doula in during the second half of the pregnancy, for somewhere between one and three prenatal visits. These visits usually occur in your home and involve some education and support—some doulas even offer specific services such as natural childbirth classes or breastfeeding education and support. This is a time for the doula to really understand your birth preferences and goals and help you develop a plan to achieve them. Your doula may accompany you to one or more of your midwife visits so that the doula and midwife get a chance to meet each other. Different practitioners do things in different ways, so you'll want to talk with your doula about how they personally work.

Natural Nutrition

One important way to help ensure a healthy pregnancy is through nutrition. Whole grains, lean protein, vegetables, and fruits should be the staples of your diet. Proteins are the building blocks of human bodies, and you're literally growing a tiny human, so your protein intake will often need to be adjusted up. (If you're a vegetarian or vegan, this doesn't mean you have to start eating meat. Just make sure you maintain good protein sources.)

Processed and fast foods are often high in sodium and lack quality vitamins and minerals, so they should be limited or avoided. There is no known safe amount of alcohol consumption during pregnancy, so it is best to avoid all alcoholic beverages. As for other food restrictions you may hear about, such as fish or cheese, the details vary, so it's best to speak with your midwife if you have any concerns about a particular food.

At the same time, it's good to remember that you're not expected to have a 100 percent perfect diet all the time. I generally recommend a goal of 80 percent good, high-quality choices and 20 percent less-than-perfect choices. For example, while you shouldn't eat french fries on a regular basis, you can save them for an occasional treat.

There's an old saying that when you're pregnant, you're "eating for two," but that's not quite true. Pregnancy only requires you to consume an additional 300 calories on top of your regular pre-pregnancy daily intake. But because of the "eating for two" myth, many pregnant people overeat. Consuming extra calories doesn't offer any advantages for your pregnancy and could actually have a negative impact if it involves low-quality foods. If you're concerned about your diet, consult with your midwife, who will typically have training and knowledge about nutrition and can offer guidance that's individually tailored to your lifestyle and dietary preferences or requirements.

You will, of course, gain weight as your pregnancy progresses—not just from the baby inside you but also from the placenta, the amniotic fluid, and your blood volume, which will increase by 50 percent over the first half of your pregnancy. Being mindful of your diet can help ensure that you gain an appropriate amount of weight, which is different for every individual and can best be determined with your midwife.

Another crucial aspect of this equation is your activity level. Remember that labor and birth are physically demanding events, and being active during your pregnancy will help you maintain your endurance and stamina. This does not mean that you need to become an elite athlete; it simply means being active on a regular basis. Generally, I recommend walking, jogging, or swimming for 30 minutes at a time, four or five days per week. Be sure to discuss this with your midwife, as they'll tailor this recommendation to your particular situation.

Additionally, pregnant people should take a daily vitamin designed specifically for prenatal needs. Your midwife will discuss vitamins and supplements with you and recommend specific ones based on your needs.

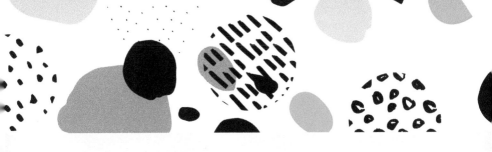

Birth Story: DOULAS AND DEPLOYMENT

Susan was pregnant with her second baby. She and her wife, Julie, had planned this new addition with joy and love, and the soon-to-be big sister couldn't have been happier to be getting a little brother. But Julie was in the military, and during the third trimester, she found out that she'd be deployed during the weeks around Susan's due date. Of course, this was difficult news. Military families are well prepared for these realities, but that doesn't make them any easier.

We needed to find a way to help Susan and her daughter feel supported, and quickly. Knowing that her family was well cared for would also help Julie focus on her work. I reached out to local doula contacts, and we found a wonderful labor doula to be with Susan during her birth process. On top of that, we found a sibling doula to help with their daughter. Sibling doulas are trained specifically to be present for children at births, supporting them with undivided attention while the parents are busy with the work of labor.

When Susan's labor started, she came to the birth center with her daughter and both doulas. We had pictures of Julie for Susan to focus on as well as a special musical playlist that Julie had prepared for Susan. Miraculously, Julie was able to call in on the phone! We didn't know where she was in the world, but she was able to join in and offer her love. It was a powerful and magical birth—not the way anyone had first envisioned it, but no less special. Surrounded by love and support, Susan gracefully welcomed her son to the world.

Dealing with the Discomforts of Pregnancy

Midwives are experts in dealing with the common discomforts of pregnancy. They're trained to know when an issue is serious and requires more significant intervention (or even referral to a different kind of provider). Depending on the type of midwife you're seeing, they may recommend alternative or natural remedies, or they may offer more medical interventions and prescriptions. Some midwives are comfortable with all these choices. There are no one-size-fits-all remedies, so your midwife will help guide you toward whatever's most appropriate for you.

The important thing is to keep your midwife aware of how you're feeling and informed about any uncomfortable symptoms you're experiencing. Pregnancy is a time of massive change, and dealing with symptoms you've never had before can be scary. Working with your midwife to understand why they occur and to try various comfort measures can help alleviate any stress or worry you may have.

Here are a few of the most common discomforts and some possible ways to help. Of course, this does not replace the advice of your own midwife, who knows your individual situation best.

MORNING SICKNESS

One of the most common and notorious complaints of early pregnancy is morning sickness, a form of nausea that may or may not also include vomiting. Despite its name, it can happen at any time of the day. We don't know exactly what causes morning sickness, also known as "nausea and vomiting of pregnancy" or NVP, but it likely has something to do with the hormonal shifts that take place during pregnancy.

There are several ways to lessen the effects of morning sickness. One is eating small, protein-filled meals and snacks frequently throughout the day. I highly recommend raw almonds and suggest keeping them around to snack on. It can be helpful to keep some by your bed and eat a couple before getting up in the morning. Sour foods can be beneficial for some people as well—think candied ginger, lemon drops, and fresh pickles. You can also try basic acupressure through commercially available wristbands designed to help alleviate motion sickness.

If these methods don't offer enough relief, I recommend an over-the-counter supplement regimen of vitamin B_6 as well as the sleep aid Unisom before bed. Thankfully, for most individuals, morning sickness peaks in severity between 8 and 10 weeks and resolves by the end of the first trimester. (For information about a more serious version of this condition, hyperemesis gravidarum, see page 66.)

HEARTBURN

Another frequent pregnancy complaint is heartburn. Prior to my own pregnancy, I had never experienced it, but during my first pregnancy, boy oh boy—suddenly I understood why every third commercial on TV was for heartburn remedies! Heartburn can present in a few ways, but typically it's an intense burning sensation in the center of your chest or the back of your throat, which may be accompanied by uncomfortable burping. Pregnancy-related heartburn typically happens because the hormone progesterone causes the sphincter at the top of the stomach to loosen, which allows stomach acid to "reflux," or flow upward into the esophagus (the tube that connects your throat to your stomach).

For clients with heartburn, I recommend eating small frequent meals and avoiding certain herbs in the mint family, which can make the problem worse. An easy home remedy that many of my clients find effective is to drink a couple tablespoons of apple cider vinegar each morning. Over-the-counter chewable calcium tablets and/or papaya-enzyme tablets can be helpful, too.

If the heartburn is severe, other causes have been ruled out, and the remedies listed previously don't give any relief, you can also try over-the-counter stomach-acid-reducing tablets. And if *those* medications don't work, there are prescription-strength versions that many midwives can write a prescription for. Note that it's important to discuss heartburn with your provider; it's usually benign, but it can also be a symptom of serious conditions.

HEMORRHOIDS

Many pregnant people will experience hemorrhoids, which are essentially large varicose veins that occur at the anus. If you have hemorrhoids, you might feel a burning and/or itchy sensation around your anus and possibly bleed bright red blood. Hemorrhoids often show up in the third trimester, as the weight of the pregnant uterus applies pressure to the pelvis. The good news is that most of the time they remain relatively small and manageable.

It's critical to avoid constipation, which can both create hemorrhoids and make preexisting ones worse. Stay regular by drinking plenty of fluids, eating plenty of fiber, and exercising. If you're experiencing discomfort from hemorrhoids, you can try this easy, inexpensive, and effective home remedy for inflammation: Grate a russet potato, wrap a small handful in cheesecloth, and apply it to the hemorrhoid(s) two to three times per day, for about 15 minutes at a time. (Unfortunately, you can't grate the potato ahead of time—it has to be freshly grated for each application.) You can also try over-the-counter witch-hazel pads. If none of that works, your midwife may recommend prescription-strength suppositories or refer you to a proctologist, who specializes in this area of the body.

Serious Complications during Pregnancy

In healthy folks with normal pregnancies, serious complications are rare. However, they can happen to anyone, so it's important to discuss any concerns with your midwife. One benefit of regular prenatal care with a competent provider is that if any complications do arise, they can usually be recognized early and addressed quickly.

Depending on the specific complication and the type of midwife you're seeing, they may need to co-manage your care with a physician or completely transfer your care to them. If you had been planning a birth at home or at a freestanding birth center, you may need to move into a hospital instead. Through all of this, your midwife will get your informed consent at every step and provide support and education on all the recommendations.

There are a few complications that are more common than others. It's important to feel informed about them, but also know that knowledge does not replace the care of your midwife, who you should always keep informed of any concerning symptoms you may experience.

HYPEREMESIS GRAVIDARUM

Earlier, we discussed simple morning sickness, or NVP, which can usually be relieved with basic comfort measures and ends with the first trimester. Normal morning sickness involves nausea and occasional vomiting, but it doesn't dehydrate you or prevent you from eating enough food or gaining the appropriate amount of weight. Hyperemesis gravidarum (HG) is a completely different complication. People with HG are plagued by severe nausea and persistent, significant vomiting. They typically become dehydrated and malnourished, to the point that they require IV infusions of fluids and nutrients.

HG is a serious complication that requires medical management, prescription medications, and close monitoring of fetal growth. But don't panic—if you're seeing a certified nurse midwife (CNM), they'll likely be able to prescribe these medications and continue to manage your care while consulting with a physician. If you're seeing another type of midwife, they may need to transfer your care over to a physician. Either way, they'll support you and offer education and resources on HG and how to cope with the diagnosis.

BLEEDING

Bleeding during pregnancy can be a frightening experience, but it's not always a cause for concern. Many women have some light pink or dark brown "spotting" (minor vaginal bleeding) in the first trimester. If this spotting is minimal and doesn't involve any uterine cramping, it's usually not a sign of complications—though you should discuss it with your midwife. You should immediately call your midwife if you see bright red bleeding, regardless of how far along you are. If this happens in the second or third trimester, it can be a sign of complications with your placenta and warrants investigation.

If your midwife works in a hospital, they'll likely have you meet them there for a full evaluation, with or without a physician consult. If your midwife doesn't work in a hospital, they'll probably still have you go to the hospital, but a consulting physician will perform the evaluation. Either way, your midwife will be there to offer support and guidance through this experience.

HIGH BLOOD PRESSURE

During pregnancy, your blood pressure will typically remain at your normal baseline or even go down a bit. However, approximately 5 to 8 percent of pregnant people experience an increase in blood pressure. High blood pressure, or hypertension, related to pregnancy is a potentially life-threatening complication that should be taken very seriously. If not properly treated, it can turn into a condition called preeclampsia, which can lead to seizures and strokes if you don't receive medical attention.

Your midwife will closely monitor your blood pressure throughout the pregnancy at each prenatal visit, keeping an eye out for other possible hypertension symptoms such as severe headaches, changes in your vision, significant heartburn, and new nausea and vomiting beginning in the third trimester. If you develop hypertension or preeclampsia, your midwife will consult with a physician, and you'll need to plan a hospital birth. Depending on how far along you are in the pregnancy, it may be necessary to immediately induce your labor. Your midwife should explain everything to you and will help support you through this process. If your midwife is a CNM and can attend your birth in a hospital, they may be able to stay involved with your care and co-manage with a physician.

WHEN TO CALL THE MIDWIFE

If you have a healthy pregnancy, there will likely be no reason to place an immediate call to your midwife until you begin labor. However, if you experience any of these three problems, you should call your midwife ASAP and make a plan about how to proceed.

1. **Decreased fetal movement.** If, in the third trimester, you have any concerns about the pattern and strength of how the baby is moving, call your midwife.

2. **Bright red vaginal bleeding.** If you experience heavy bleeding like a menstrual period, get in touch with your midwife immediately.

3. **Water breaking.** If you think your water may have broken or if it clearly has broken, pick up the phone and call your midwife right away.

Losing the Pregnancy

As we just discussed, many women may experience some light spotting in the first trimester, and this can be normal. Unfortunately, sometimes first-trimester bleeding along with uterine cramping can be a sign of a miscarriage. Miscarriage is the loss of a pregnancy, usually in the first trimester. It is very important to remember that this is almost never the fault of the pregnant person. Usually, miscarriage occurs because the fetus just wasn't developing normally. Sadly, once a miscarriage has begun, there is no way to stop it. From a physical standpoint, most miscarriages will happen on their own, but you should always notify your midwife of heavy bleeding so they can perform an exam and be certain you don't need medical intervention.

Miscarriage is not the only way people lose pregnancies. Some pregnant people discover several weeks or months in that their pregnancy is ectopic. An ectopic pregnancy happens when a fertilized egg implants somewhere outside the uterus, usually in one of the fallopian tubes. It's rare, but when it does happen, it is life-threatening for the pregnant person. A fallopian tube is not able to accommodate or nourish an embryo the way a uterus is, and as the pregnancy grows, the fallopian tube can rupture, leading to significant internal bleeding.

Whenever a pregnant person experiences pain and bleeding in the first trimester, they need to immediately call a medical professional, who can check to see if they have an ectopic pregnancy. For this reason, you must always notify your midwife if you have these symptoms. Your midwife will need to perform blood work and an ultrasound or refer you to a physician who can. If your practitioners find that your pregnancy is ectopic, you'll need immediate medical intervention.

To be clear, ectopic pregnancies cannot and will not grow to become a healthy baby, and the embryo can't be moved from the fallopian tube to the uterus. The only option is to save the life of the pregnant person by ending the pregnancy. If an ectopic pregnancy is diagnosed early enough, it may be treatable with medication alone. If it is diagnosed later, the pregnant person will need to undergo a surgical procedure to remove the embryo.

Losing a pregnancy is emotionally and psychologically complicated, but you're not alone. About 10 to 20 percent of recognized pregnancies end in miscarriage. Other women in your personal community have likely been through the same experience and can help support you. Additionally, your midwife will be present and available to help you cope and answer your questions. They will likely have a list of local resources and support groups if you want more structured support.

It's important to take some time to heal both physically and emotionally after this loss. There is no quick fix, and treating yourself with grace and patience while allowing yourself to feel all the emotions you experience will be helpful. You may feel sad, angry, or confused—or all of these at the same time. You may need to talk about it a lot, or you may not want to talk about it at all. There is no right or wrong way to feel.

Partners in Pregnancy

Perhaps the most important member of your birth team other than you is your partner. In most cases, they'll be intimately involved in your pregnancy and will spend the most time with you in the months leading up to your birth. If you don't have a partner or your partner is not able to be with you physically, it will be helpful to identify a person from your family or community who can partially fill this role. If you don't have someone like this, a doula can be a helpful resource.

Your partner can and should be a valuable source of support on a day-to-day basis. For example, they might help with your nutrition and exercise goals by working on meal planning and exercising with you. They can do simple household tasks that may become more challenging for you as the pregnancy progresses. And never underestimate the healing power of a good foot or shoulder massage!

It's helpful for your partner to accompany you to at least some of your prenatal appointments with the midwife. Some partners are able to attend all the visits, and some are only able to attend a few. We all have busy lives and schedules, and the demands of work are real, so if your partner can't be at every appointment, that's okay. Your midwife will understand, and no one will hold it against you or them.

For big-picture issues like creating your birth plan, your partner's involvement is crucial. They know you well and can support you in making the choices that best fit you and your goals. It's also a good way for them to be involved with and included in your pregnancy. Working on baby planning is a great way to encourage communication and connection between the two of you. Researching all the latest and greatest baby gear, finding a pediatrician, choosing a name ... these are all necessary steps, and your partner can and should be an integral part of these decisions.

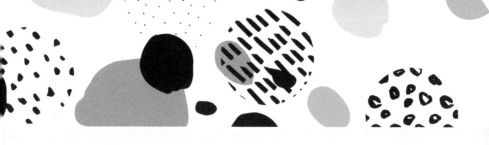

Birth Story:
NOT THE WAY SHE PLANNED IT

Estela and her partner had done all the "right" things when preparing for their first child. She had some of the normal pregnancy complaints—morning sickness in the first weeks and some difficulty sleeping as her baby grew—but nothing alarming. Then, at her 38-week prenatal exam, we discovered her blood pressure had increased dramatically from her normal baseline. She also reported severe headaches over the preceding few days. We drew some blood, collected a urine sample, and did some tests. The tests showed that the baby was fine— but Estela had developed preeclampsia. At 38 weeks, with that diagnosis, the current recommendation is to induce labor and have a baby. We explained this to Estela and her partner, answering all their questions and giving them lots of support.

They gave consent to go to the hospital and induce labor. They were of course disappointed in this sudden turn of events, but we tried to focus on the positive: We were looking forward to a birthday! During the course of her labor, Estela's blood pressure spiked to dangerously high levels that we had to treat with IV medications. (One of our physician partners was present to help if needed.)

With each new obstacle, Estela would take deep breaths, talk with her partner, and then gracefully accept the new recommendations. Her all-natural, unmedicated birth plan had to be completely tossed out the window, but she still had

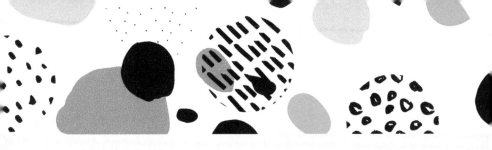

her midwife and her family at her side. We made sure she was thoroughly informed and involved in all decisions, supporting her through all the changes. Eventually, she gave birth to her son—not in the way she had envisioned but in the way he needed—and the room held just as much love and joy as it does at any birth. Thankfully, after the birth, her blood pressure came back down, and her other symptoms began to stabilize. Both Estela and her baby had normal recoveries and went on to thrive.

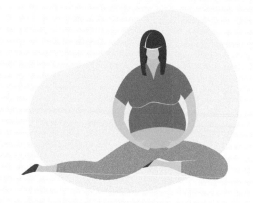

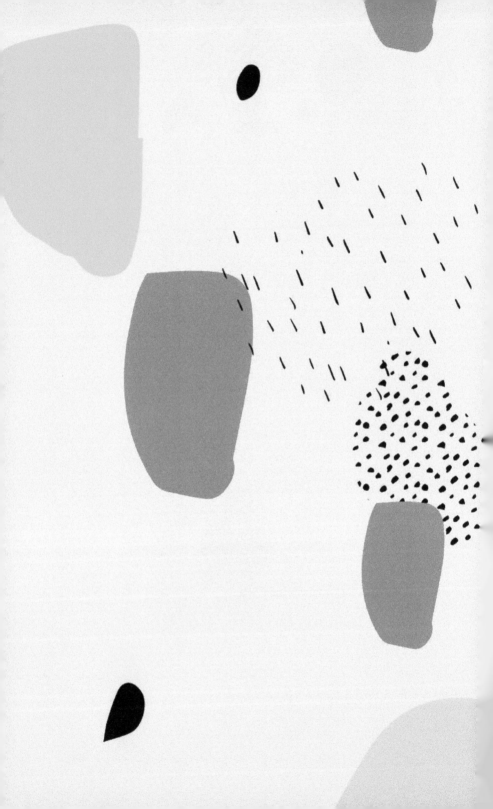

CHAPTER 4

Preparing for Childbirth

Preparing for the big day can be both exciting and overwhelming! Looking at all the things you have to do can feel intimidating, but remember that you don't have to do everything at once. Your midwife will be an excellent resource to help you figure out what to focus on and when. This chapter will also help you break the preparation list down into smaller, more manageable tasks.

Birth Plan Basics

At its most basic, a birth plan is just that: a plan for you and your birth team to follow when you're giving birth. It might include information like where you want to give birth, who you want to have present, and what should happen if anything unexpected occurs. Here are some questions that often come up about birth plans.

Why create a birth plan? Birth plans can be a valuable part of the preparation process as you learn about all your options, decide which ones best fit your needs and desires, and communicate your plans to your birth team. The process of educating yourself is always valuable, no matter what kind of birth you're having. Remember that plans can change, and you may end up needing to give birth in a setting you didn't expect. In these cases, it's incredibly helpful to have tools to help you communicate with new providers and staff in a potentially stressful situation.

At what point in the pregnancy do you typically create a birth plan? You can start the informal process of gathering resources right away. People usually start formally outlining and preparing the plan as they enter the third trimester.

Who should be involved in creating your birth plan? What role does the midwife play? The most important people are you and your partner. You are the ones who will be experiencing this process, so your opinions matter most. Stand firm and confident in your educated decisions. However, it's also critical to involve your midwife so they know your desires and can answer any questions you have about your options. For example, if you're planning a hospital birth, what are the policies that may affect your birth plans? Do they require certain types of fetal monitoring? What are their policies on eating and drinking in labor? These are important questions as you craft your birth plan, and your midwife will be able to help answer them.

What role does the doula play? Doulas can also be great resources for education and support. Even if a doula isn't involved in creating a birth plan, they should have access to the finalized version so they know your choices.

Once you've created the birth plan, is it set in stone, or can it change? When it comes to labor and birth, the name of the game must always be flexibility and adaptation. Things can and do change, and we need to remain open to the process. Your midwife will help guard your most important wishes and ensure that you stay as close to the plan as possible.

How long should a birth plan be? I highly recommend keeping it to one page, especially if you're planning a hospital birth. Bulleted lists with graphics can be very helpful—for example, a simple picture of an apple and a water drop if you want to be able to eat and drink freely. Hospital staff have a lot of paperwork to keep track of, so you want your birth plan to communicate your core desires in an easy-to-read, straightforward manner. A plan that is multiple pages long can easily get lost in translation.

What if your provider and chosen place of birth don't agree with what is outlined on your birth plan? Then you may need to consider making some changes, especially if the parts of the plan that they have issues with are the parts that are most essential to you and your partner. It may take some serious effort on your part, but it's possible to change providers or birth locations, even late in the process. Going through the plan with your provider early can help identify any concerns and areas to discuss further while giving you time to make alternate choices if necessary.

When discussing birth plans, it's important to acknowledge that we don't always have control over everything that happens in labor and birth, so we have to be open to making adjustments and changes. I often describe it to clients like this: You are the director of a play. You cast the actors (your partner, your midwife), pick the setting (home, birth center, or hospital), and choose the props and wardrobe. You oversee rehearsals by taking classes, reading books, and putting together a birth plan. But ultimately, the performance is out of your control. You can do everything correctly and still have a completely different experience than you hoped for. All the planning and education in the world can't guarantee the birth of your dreams. This can be difficult to accept, but talking about it with your midwife can alleviate some of the inherent stress.

Creating Your Birth Plan

A good birth plan will be based on the research you've done on your own and with your birth team. What you choose to include is up to you, but here are some of the issues that are important to consider.

Who will be present? Clarify who's on your birth team by name. This is especially important if you're planning a hospital birth or if you have to transfer to a hospital during your labor. In those cases, you'll be encountering many people you've never met, so having a way to identify your team can be critical. If possible, include photos of the key players like your partner, midwife, and doula. Also list the names of friends and family members you may want nearby and your birth photographer if you're using one. (Some hospitals may have restrictions on the presence of photographers, so be sure to research this beforehand.)

If you have other children, where will they be? Including children in the process can be a beautiful experience and can help with sibling bonding. If you do decide to include other children, it's important to use age-appropriate education to prepare them ahead of time and to plan on having a support person present for them if they need to leave the birth space. (Some hospitals may have restrictions on small children being present, so be sure to research this beforehand as well.)

How do you want to engage your senses? What do you want to see? Are there special photographs, colors, or focal points you want to include in the space? What do you want to smell? Are there scents that help you relax and/or wake up? Are there odors you really don't like that should be avoided? Is there any special music you want to hear? (I always recommend two playlists: one filled with relaxing music and one with music that helps wake you up and get the juices flowing.) Or would you prefer it to be quiet? What do you want to feel on your skin? What clothes will you wear? Do you want to be touched? Is massage helpful for you?

What are your pain management goals? Do you want to be able to move freely? Are you planning an unmedicated birth? If pain medication becomes necessary, what types are you open to? Many families who are planning an unmedicated birth will choose a word or phrase that the laboring person can use to communicate that the plan has changed and they truly want pain medication.

What do you want to happen at the moment of birth? What body positions would you like to be able to use? Common birth positions include being on your hands and knees, lying on your side, and squatting. Do you want immediate skin-to-skin contact with the baby? Are you planning delayed, or physiologic, cord clamping? (For more information, see page 118.) And when it's time to cut the cord, who will do that?

Do you want to keep the placenta? Though most families don't keep the placenta, some opt to hold on to it after the birth. In general, it's easier to keep the placenta if you're giving birth at home or in a birth center. If you give birth in a hospital, it may require some extra planning, coordination, and signing of forms. Some cultures have specific rituals that dictate what happens to the placenta, like burying it. Other people may want to practice "placentophagy," which means eating the placenta—drinking it as part of a smoothie, dehydrating it and consuming it in pill form, or ingesting it in various other ways. Some believe placentophagy has benefits like decreasing overall blood loss and protecting against postpartum depression, though these benefits have not been proven by research. Ingesting the placenta can be safe and hygienic if the person preparing it follows safe practices. If you want to keep your placenta, you should thoroughly discuss your plans with your midwife ahead of time.

What if there's a change in plans? If an unplanned cesarean section becomes necessary, who do you want in the operating room with you? Typically, for safety, the number of support people will be limited to one or two. Designate ahead of time who that will be.

What will initial baby care be like? Who will touch the baby? Should medications and bathing be delayed until after breastfeeding has happened? Where do you want the baby to be? For example, if you're planning a hospital birth, does the hospital have a separate nursery they'll take the baby to? And if so, who will go with the baby? (In a home or birth-center birth, the baby will automatically remain with the parents the entire time.)

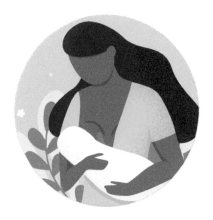

Birth Plan Template

If you need a good starting place, this template will help you begin to write your own birth plan.

BIRTH PLAN FOR THE ________________ FAMILY

The Birth Team: Clearly identify your team by name and what their role is. Provide small pictures in the final version of the plan if possible.

Labor Preferences: How do you want your labor to look and feel? Be specific and clear about what you want and how you've prepared for it.

Pain Management: Delineate your goals, but also discuss how to make adjustments if necessary. Go over what kind of support and techniques do or don't work for you.

_____

_____

_____

_____

_____

Moment of Birth: Who will be present? What will happen with the baby if all is well? What do you request if interventions become necessary?

_____

_____

_____

_____

_____

Placenta Preferences: Do you plan to keep the placenta? If so, do you plant to ingest it?

_____

_____

_____

continued

Change of Plans: If you end up needing a cesarean section or other unexpected intervention, how would you like this to be handled? Who will be with you, and who will be with the baby? Remember that changes can happen quickly during labor.

_____

_____

_____

_____

_____

_____

Baby Care: Be sure to know the policies ahead of time and discuss them with your midwife. Have a plan for the likely event that all will go well, but also note what your preferences are if intervention is needed.

_____

_____

_____

_____

_____

_____

Sample Birth Plan

To give you an idea of what a finished birth plan might look like, here's a sample birth plan for the fictional Jones family.

BIRTH PLAN FOR THE JONES FAMILY AT PEACE VALLEY HOSPITAL

The Birth Team: **The birthing person is Sara, her partner is Tom, and our midwife is Janelle. We'll also have with us a doula named Max, as well as Beth, a photographer who will be shooting stills and video. We do not plan on any other support people or guests joining us.**

Labor Preferences: **Sara wants to be free to move with her labor, declines intravenous access, and will drink fluids and eat snacks. Sara's partner and doula will provide physical hands-on support with the guidance of their midwife. She has music to listen to and will play it in the room. Sara prefers the scent of lavender and will request it if she desires. Please avoid any mint essential oils.**

Pain Management: **We prefer an unmedicated birth and have prepared well for this goal. We plan to use positional changes, massage, and hydrotherapy for comfort. If Sara decides she wants to try using nitrous oxide, she will ask for**

continued

it. If an epidural becomes necessary or recommended, Sara and Tom would like a full explanation and consent process and for Tom to remain with her through the process.

Moment of Birth: Sara would like to give birth in the position that feels best to her at that time. Sara declines routine episiotomy. If our midwife thinks one is necessary, she will explain why and ask for permission. If possible, Tom would like to help the midwife with catching our baby. We prefer for the baby to be placed directly skin to skin with Sara. We plan to do delayed cord clamping and have discussed this with our midwife. We request that the room remain as quiet as possible, without extra people, unless they're needed in the event of an emergency.

Placenta Preferences: We do not plan to keep the placenta.

Change of Plans: If a cesarean section becomes necessary or recommended, Sara wants Tom to accompany her to the operating room. If possible, we would also like the photographer to join us. If there needs to be a separation of Sara and the baby, Tom will stay with the baby, and our doula will remain with Sara.

Baby Care: We request that, as long as everyone is healthy, Sara and Tom be the primary people to touch the baby in the first hour. Baby will remain skin to skin until after breastfeeding has been established. After that, we will allow the baby to be weighed and examined, in our presence. We plan to delay the first bath for 24 hours. Before any routine medications are administered, Sara and Tom will be informed and, after a full explanation, may choose to decline.

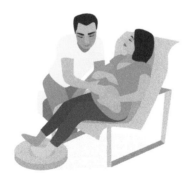

Taking Classes

Education is a key step in preparing for childbirth, one of the most physically demanding and emotionally charged events that humans experience. For most people, their own labor and birth will be the first one they witness and participate in, so it's critical to prepare yourself and your birth partner. Classes on topics like childbirth preparation and newborn care will help.

Your midwife will know the available courses in your specific area, who the teachers are, and which ones are the best. Some midwives with extra training even offer these courses themselves.

For first-time parents, I recommend taking three types of classes: childbirth preparation, breast/chest feeding, and newborn care.

CHILDBIRTH PREPARATION CLASSES

This should be a comprehensive course that meets multiple times. You'll learn all about each of the stages of labor and birth as well as coping techniques and strategies to move though each phase. This class should also inform you about potential complications, so that if you end up experiencing one, you'll have a basic understanding of what's happening and won't feel as scared. These classes come in many different styles and philosophies, and it's important to choose one that fits your and your partner's learning styles. This course is an investment in all your plans, so be thoughtful about the decision.

BREAST/CHEST FEEDING CLASSES

If you plan to breastfeed/chest feed (some people who give birth prefer the term "chest feeding" instead of "breastfeeding," especially if they're transgender or nonbinary), it's critical to prepare yourself and your partner ahead of the birth. It comes easily to some, but for many others, it requires some extra work. Unfortunately, in our current culture, most of us don't grow up with much exposure to lactation. A good class will give you the skills and knowledge you need to support this choice. It's also helpful to identify resources and community before there are any issues and put plans in place to respond to possible common hurdles. (For more information, see page 141.)

NEWBORN CARE CLASSES

Being the primary care provider for an infant is challenging! It's the best job in the world and the hardest, all rolled into one messy bundle. Learning the basics ahead of time can alleviate some of the stress and pressure. Knowing what's normal and what's abnormal is extremely helpful. I also highly recommend an infant first aid and CPR class.

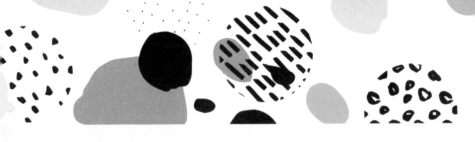

Birth Story: OTHER PLANS

Saba and Adam were seasoned parents. They already had three beautiful daughters and were preparing to welcome their first son. Their other children had all made their arrivals before their actual due dates, but this little boy had other ideas. Saba's due date came and went. At one week past, we did some extra testing to be sure they were both healthy. They were. Then we had a good long talk about expectations, letting go, and acknowledging that we didn't have control over when this birthday would happen.

Then, 10 days after her due date, Saba called in labor. The catch? She was home alone. It was the middle of the day. Her daughters were with their nanny. Adam was over 45 minutes away at work—and he had the birth kit in his car. To top it all off, this baby had decided he was now coming fast. The nanny agreed to keep the kids longer, Adam left work to head for the birth center, and Saba called her neighbor for a ride. I got the birth center ready to welcome everyone.

Saba arrived first, in active labor but holding herself back. The brain is powerful and can have a huge impact on labor. Her husband had not arrived yet, and she would not have this baby without him! When he did walk in, she let out a deep sigh, locked eyes with him, and thirty minutes later, while squatting by the birth pool, welcomed her sweet baby boy into their arms. We then tucked them into bed and had a laugh about how none of our expectations matter when a baby has other plans.

Assembling Your Birth Kit

Whether you plan to give birth at home, at a birth center, or in a hospital, you'll need to have certain supplies on hand. It's a good idea to assemble these items ahead of time so you won't be caught by surprise when you need them.

HOME BIRTH KIT

Choosing to give birth at home is a powerful option—and the one that will require the most planning on your part. Your midwife will be very involved in educating you and your birth team on what materials you'll need.

In general, you'll want to keep the birth space tidy during the last few weeks of your pregnancy. Pay attention to the weather and the entrance to your home. Will the midwife have a place to park? Does the sidewalk need to be shoveled? These seemingly mundane things will be important on the big day.

Your midwife will bring all the necessary safety equipment and supplies, including the instruments necessary to listen to your baby during labor, monitor your vital signs, and manage the birth itself. They'll also bring emergency equipment in the rare event that it's needed. Your midwife will also give *you* a list of items to prepare and have ready ahead of time. Some midwives work with birth-supply companies and have custom birth kits designed specifically for them that contain most of the supplies they recommend you have on hand. Others will give you a detailed list of things to gather. Your individual midwife will go over their system and preferences with you one-on-one.

Some standard items that most midwives will request or recommend you have on hand are:

- Plenty of clean towels, blankets, and a baby hat.

- Food for both the laboring person and the support team.

- Underpads (disposable or reusable). These large, absorbent pads are placed under the laboring person to help catch fluids both during the labor and after the birth.

- Sanitary pads for your postpartum bleeding. I highly recommend using an adult diaper for the first couple of days. It may sound silly, but the bleeding can be like a heavy period, and you'll be busy with a newborn.

- Peri bottle. This is a small, squeezable water bottle with a nozzle that allows you to irrigate your perineum before and after you pee.

- A waterproof mattress bag or cover for your bed to protect it from blood and fluids.

In general, since you're at home, you'll already have access to all your routine comfort items—your own clothing, hygiene products, kitchen, bathroom, etc. Measures like aromatherapy and music are easy to accommodate and plan for in your own home as well. Plus you get to be in control of who is present. Your midwife will help you review your plans for visitors and family members.

Here are some tools you may wish to make use of while you're in labor. Birth centers and some hospitals will have this equipment, but if you're planning a home birth, you'll want to ask your midwife about acquiring them.

A **birthing ball** is a typical exercise ball, like you'd find at the gym. It can be very helpful to gently bounce on one during contractions or to lean on it in certain birth positions. A "peanut ball" is a more specialized birth ball that looks (not surprisingly) like a large peanut. This can also be helpful if your midwife has one.

A **birthing stool** is a horseshoe-shaped stool you can sit on while in labor. The shape makes it easier for the baby to come out and lets the midwife access the process more easily. Your midwife will likely have one of these, but it's a good idea to confirm that with them beforehand.

A **birthing pool** can be any sanitary pool of warm water. At home, people often use their bathtub. There are also specialized inflatable or collapsible birth pools, which a midwife may bring to your house or have you order yourself. One thing that sets birth centers (and some hospitals) apart is that they have bigger, deeper, permanent birthing pools.

HOSPITAL BIRTH KIT

If you're planning a hospital birth with a midwife, you won't be required to prepare as many supplies, but you'll still need to communicate with your midwife about the situation. Of course, the hospital will have all the necessary medical supplies and equipment for the midwife to access, as well as postpartum supplies like peri bottles and sanitary pads. Your midwife will help you determine what you're expected to bring—or not bring—with you. For example, does the hospital encourage laboring people to eat and drink? If so, can you bring in your own food? Are you allowed to bring in items like candles and aromatherapy supplies? What are the hospital's policies on visitors? These are important topics to discuss and plan for ahead of time with your midwife.

Think about the mundane things as well. Be sure to keep the gas tank in the car at least half full during the last few weeks of pregnancy. (A laboring person will not be happy to stop for gas in the middle of the trip!) Know where you're going, and plan out an alternate route to the hospital in case of traffic or bad weather.

Some common items to pack in your hospital birth kit are:

- Personal hygiene products like a toothbrush and toothpaste, lip balm, shampoo, and body wash. Don't forget to pack these items for your partner as well!

- A change of clothes to wear home (and, depending on the hospital policies, special clothes to labor in).

- Clothing for the baby to wear when going home.

- A car seat to take the baby home in.

- Comfort items, like a special pillow or blanket, if desired.

BIRTH-CENTER BIRTH KIT

As far as supplies go, planning a birth-center birth is similar to planning a hospital birth. The birth center will have the necessary equipment stocked and ready. Typically, birth centers will have more than one birth-room option and will note your favorite in your chart so they can prepare the space when you're on your way. The midwife will fill the birth pool, light candles, start aromatherapy, and make the space feel welcoming. As with a home birth, you'll be encouraged to eat and drink during your labor. Some birth centers will request that you bring in your own food, while others will supply the food. Birth centers will support you in including whomever you choose to be present at your birth and will accommodate your full birth team.

As with a hospital birth, be sure to plan for mundane things like gas and directions. The birth kit you'll pack will be the same as the hospital birth kit detailed previously—plus a swimsuit for the pregnant person's partner, if they're encouraged to get in the birth pool as well.

Preparing Emotionally

Pregnancy can feel like a roller coaster, full of change and big emotions. The days seem long, but the weeks fly by. For many people, the last few weeks can be the hardest. Sharing your body with another human, even though it's natural and our bodies are designed to do it, is not easy. Physically, it can become pretty uncomfortable. Sleep can be elusive, navigating your body through the world can be challenging, and your emotions can be all over the map. All of this adds up to some rough weeks. Most pregnant people will become noticeably grumpy, may cry at the drop of a hat, and will sometimes have very little patience to spare. On top of that, you may feel the need to double- and triple-check your supplies and plans. All of this can lead to some stressful days and nights.

I call it "babyitis"—the condition that afflicts us when we're so wrapped up in anxiety about the looming big event that we forget to stay in the moment and focus on the positive aspects of the experience. I encourage all my clients not to bottle up these powerful emotions but rather to feel them and let them out. Throw a temper tantrum, cry on the bathroom floor, have a screaming session. Then take some deep breaths, drink a glass of water, shake it out, and take the next step forward. All of this is normal and part of the process. Once you release the tough emotions and regather yourself, take some time to focus on you and your partner. In the first few weeks after the baby comes, you'll both be busy and sleep-deprived, so take this time to go on a nice walk in the fresh air, see a movie, or go to your favorite restaurant that isn't kid-friendly. Put some good time and memories in the bank, sleep well, and take each day as it comes.

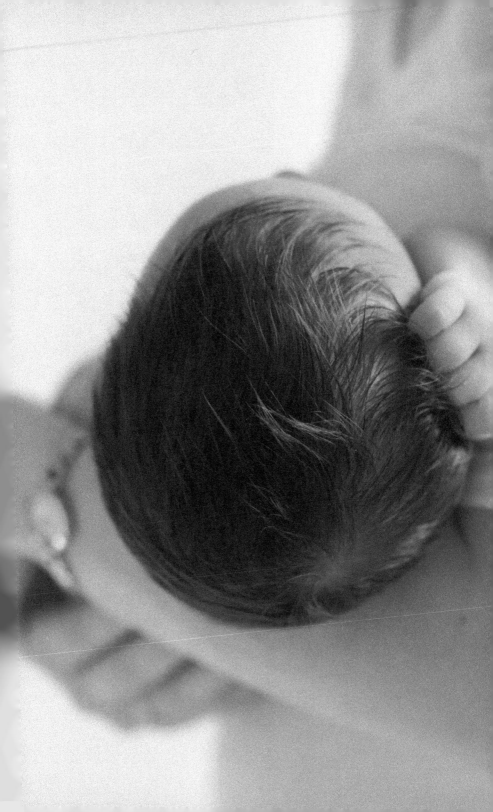

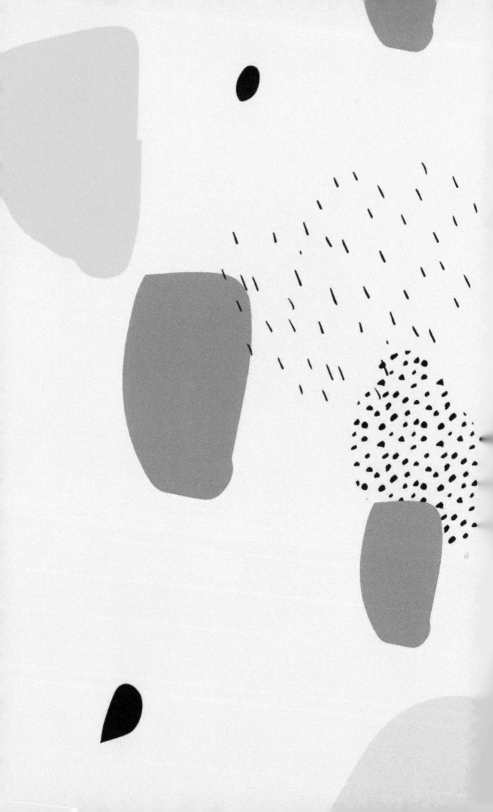

CHAPTER 5

Childbirth with a Midwife

Birth is sometimes called an everyday miracle, and once you've been part of one, you know why. You've prepared for these hours all throughout your pregnancy, but when the time finally comes, it can feel overwhelming. But don't worry. You can do this, and your midwife will be there with you to support and guide you through the process. This chapter will walk you through how that process will feel and look.

Going into Labor

As a midwife, one of the most common questions I'm asked is "What does labor feel like?" I absolutely understand the question. Childbirth is a huge unknown, one that defies description; there is truly nothing else to compare it to. Unfortunately, in our current culture, we're typically taught from a young age that it will be the most painful thing that ever happens to us. Labor is indeed hard work—quite possibly the hardest work you'll ever do. (There's a reason it's called "labor"!) But it is very doable. Your body is built to do this work, and at the end of the process, you get one of the best rewards possible.

Labor is an example of our bodies working properly—though the common media portrayal of labor as a medical procedure in a hospital makes many people believe otherwise. If you go to the dentist to have a cavity filled, there is a problem. If you break your leg or develop a kidney stone, there is a problem. The pain is a reflection of something going wrong. Labor, on the other hand, is *supposed* to happen. This is not to say that the sensations are easy or fun but rather that we need to alter our expectations and understanding of those sensations. The work of labor is allowing yourself to let go so that it can happen.

So what does labor feel like? It feels like hard work! But there's a difference between working hard and suffering. You should not suffer, and your midwife will help make sure that doesn't happen. Throughout your pregnancy, your midwife will prepare you for the start of the labor process. They will give you instructions on when, why, and how to call them when labor begins.

For most healthy, low-risk pregnant people, labor will start spontaneously sometime between 37 and 42 weeks, and there will be no intervention required. However, there are situations in which labor has to be induced, either for the health of the pregnant person or for the health of the baby. Examples of appropriate reasons to induce labor include preeclampsia or gestational hypertension (pregnancy-related high blood pressure); significantly prolonged rupture of membranes without labor starting on its own; intrauterine growth restriction (IUGR), which means the baby has stopped receiving enough nutrients and isn't growing properly; and going beyond 42 weeks without labor starting. If your midwife thinks an induction may be appropriate, they will discuss it with you in depth and answer all your questions. Depending on the particular scenario and the type of midwife, they may be able to manage this process in the hospital, or they may need to transfer your care to a physician.

The First Stage of Labor

The first stage of labor stretches from the onset of regular contractions until the time your cervix is fully dilated and you can begin pushing. Technically, this stage of labor can be divided into two distinct parts: latent labor and active labor.

LATENT LABOR

Your cervix is incredibly strong because it has to be—it holds up the weight of your pregnant uterus inside your body. The baby, the placenta, and the amniotic fluid can easily weigh well over 10 pounds, and the cervix has to bear this weight and stay closed to keep the baby from coming out too soon. So when the baby *does* need to come out, and this incredibly tough tissue needs to soften and open, it can take some time.

This is the work of latent labor. You will sometimes hear it referred to as "false" or "fake" labor, but this could not be further from the truth. It is very real and very important—it's just not active labor.

Characterized by mild to moderate irregular contractions, latent labor can take anywhere from a few hours to a few days. You're most likely to have a long latent phase if you're having your first baby, but it can also happen to women who've already given birth. You might notice that the contractions come on after the sun goes down and keep you up all night, then go away when the sun comes up. This is normal. I repeat: *This is normal*. Your body is being very smart, taking the huge task of wearing down that cervix and dividing it up into manageable bits so you can take rest breaks in between. Use those rest periods to sleep, hydrate, and eat good food. Keep your midwife in the loop and let them know what you're experiencing. They can ensure you get the rest you need in between the contractions and help you with coping mechanisms like warm Epsom salt baths, showers, herbs, essential oils, massage, or over-the-counter sleep aids.

WHAT ARE CONTRACTIONS, ANYWAY?

The uterus is made of three different muscle layers. These muscles contract and relax, just like other muscles in your body do when you walk around or pick up an item. You've probably felt your uterus contract during your period—that's what menstrual cramps are. Some people have mild, irregular contractions throughout their pregnancies. These are known as Braxton-Hicks contractions, and while they're uncomfortable, they're usually not painful. At the end of pregnancy, in labor, the contractions become more rhythmic and regular. These contractions help shorten and open the cervix during the first stage of labor and then push the baby down the birth canal in the second stage.

ACTIVE LABOR

At some point, latent labor will become active labor. The work of active labor is to let go and allow the contractions to flow. These contractions are much stronger and come in a regular pattern. They won't go away based on the time of day. Active labor takes over the whole body and mind. People who are in active labor don't care about the current realities of the world. They can't watch a TV show or participate in a discussion. They will not be distractible. People in active labor moan and might make rhythmic movements. For some people, active labor means they cannot be still; they may rock back and forth or prefer to be on all fours on the floor. Other people in active labor may require stillness in order to focus.

The same person may require movement for one contraction and then stillness for the next.

The most important thing is that the person in labor is empowered to do what feels right for them and that they have a support system in place to let the energy flow and express itself. I often tell families that you don't have to be polite in active labor. Social pleasantries need not apply. This does not mean that people in active labor can or should start ranting and raving at the people around them. But they should be encouraged to simply state what they need or what they don't like without worrying about how they sound.

WHAT TO DO DURING FIRST STAGE

This is the phase of labor when you will notify and assemble your birth team, including your midwife and your doula (if you're using one). If you've planned a home birth, they will come to you. If you've planned a birth-center or hospital birth, this is when you'll travel to that location. Active labor is also the time to start using the tools you've identified while working with your midwife to create your birth plan. In what ways have you planned to engage your senses? What do you want to see, hear, taste, and feel? Your midwife and doula will both support you and your partner with coping techniques and positional changes, making sure you drink and eat enough and that you get all the key items from your birth plan. (In a hospital setting, the doula may fulfill this role more, depending on the midwifery practice.) The midwife will also be monitoring you and the baby: taking your vital signs, listening to the baby's heartbeat, performing vaginal exams (with consent and explanation) to determine the baby's position, and monitoring the changing of your cervix.

This is a time for your partner and/or other support people to take the lead on interacting with the "outside world" so you can remain fully engaged in the labor. Your partner will be the one to do most of the talking. Your partner will also make sure your birth plan is being followed and advocate for your wishes. Of course, you're still in charge of your care, but it's helpful to have your partner assist with this. Additionally, your partner may provide direct comfort measures like rubbing your shoulders, squeezing your hips, and providing back pressure.

POTENTIAL COMPLICATIONS DURING FIRST STAGE

As I've mentioned, if you're healthy and have had a low-risk pregnancy up to this point, you'll likely remain that way throughout your labor as well. However, complications can arise, including prolonged labor without progress, which can lead to exhaustion; the baby not tolerating the labor process, as indicated by changes in their heartbeat; and issues with the placenta either not functioning properly or coming detached from the uterus too soon. This is why you made the choice to have a midwife present—so they can monitor for subtle signs and changes, recognize problems early, and react quickly to get you the help you need. If you're in the hospital, these complications may require altering or adjusting your birth plan and may also necessitate a physician becoming involved. If you're in the community birth setting (i.e., at home or in a birth center), these complications may mean that you'll have to transfer care to a hospital and possibly a physician.

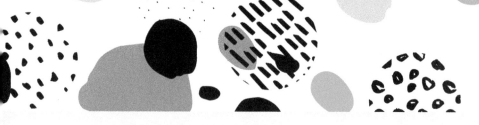

Birth Story: THE PICNIC

Kara was having her second baby and had been in active labor for about six hours. She and her partner had come to the birth center about three hours into the process, and she had quickly gone straight into the pool. Her three-year-old, who was there with a sibling doula, loved helping her drink water, gently offering the bottle and straw.

As the active phase of labor intensified, Kara worked beautifully with the sensations. She moved her body in the way that was most beneficial for her. She made low, open sounds deep in her chest. The warm water of the birth pool helped her fully relax between contractions and lifted some of the effects of gravity from her when the contractions were at their peak. Her partner was present, applying cool cloths to her forehead and shoulders and offering words of love and support. Then, just as the work reached a powerful crescendo, Kara took a deep breath, looked at me, and said she was starving. At this point, her labor stopped.

We brought in an array of food and arranged it around the pool, then sat down and passed food around to each other as if having a picnic. We chatted and laughed. Kara told a funny story. Finally, after we had all eaten, about 45 minutes after the contractions had stopped, Kara became more serious and seemed to drift out of the conversation. The contractions returned, and she began spontaneously pushing. Twenty minutes later, while still in the pool, she birthed her gorgeous new baby into the world.

The Second Stage of Labor

The first stage of labor is about letting go; the second stage is about being active. Many people struggle with the first stage and the letting-go process but feel more in control and involved with the second stage. Second stage begins with the onset of pushing and continues through to the birth of the baby. Sometimes you'll read that second stage is the time from when your cervix is fully opened until the birth of the baby, but that's not quite right. For some people, once their cervix is fully opened, their body will take a break or pause before the work of pushing begins. The work of latent and active labor can be long, and it only makes sense that our bodies may want to take a little breather before the last push to the finish line. This pause can last a few minutes up to an hour or so. Your midwife will help honor this time and will know what's normal and what requires intervention.

WHAT TO DO DURING SECOND STAGE

This is the stage when you start pushing. Some people experience involuntary, spontaneous pushing, while others may need some direction. For example, if you're in a hospital and have an epidural, coaching may be required, whereas if you're having an unmedicated birth, you're more likely to have spontaneous pushing that doesn't require a lot of direction. The pushing phase of labor can last from only a few minutes up to three or four hours. The length often depends on the position of the baby, whether it's your first baby, and whether you've had an epidural.

As you push, there will be a strong sensation of pressure. This pressure is often felt in the rectum—in fact, it can sometimes feel like your vagina is not involved and everything is happening in your bottom. This is normal. As the baby puts increasing pressure on the pelvis, the nerves in the rectum are stimulated. It is very common for people to pass stool (poop) when pushing. While this may sound scary and embarrassing, it's actually very normal. Your birth team will discreetly take care of it without drawing attention to it. As a midwife, I actually get happy when a client starts passing stool because it means they're effectively pushing and will soon have a baby!

WHAT YOUR BIRTH TEAM DOES DURING SECOND STAGE

Your midwife will be monitoring your progress, keeping an eye on your vital signs, and listening to the baby's heartbeat. They'll help manage the process, encourage and support you, suggest different positions, and make sure you and the baby remain healthy. Your doula will be there to offer support as well as to assist with positioning and other comfort measures. Your partner will help with comfort measures, too. If your partner wants to catch the baby, your midwife can help guide them to do so. Some partners want to stay up by your head with you, not seeing everything that's happening, and that's fine, too. There is no right or wrong way for your partner to be involved, as long as you're both comfortable with their role.

POTENTIAL COMPLICATIONS DURING SECOND STAGE

Complications in healthy labors are rare in the second stage, but they can happen. Examples include fetal intolerance to pushing, as indicated by the baby's heartbeat; prolonged pushing with little or no descent of the baby (which may require a physician to use forceps or a vacuum to assist with the delivery); and a rare condition called cephalopelvic disproportion (CPD), which is a fancy way of saying the baby's head is too large to fit through the mother's pelvis and a cesarean birth will be required. It is your midwife's job to monitor for any complications that can occur. If one does happen, they'll be able to recognize it and respond accordingly by transferring you to a hospital and/or calling in a physician.

MIDWIFE AS LIFEGUARD

If you've had a healthy, low-risk pregnancy, your labor and birth will likely occur without any emergencies. When we look at national data from freestanding birth centers, once someone is admitted in labor, their risk of an emergency complication is approximately 1 percent—and even less than 1 percent for the newborn. However, there are rare emergencies that can happen.

Midwives are kind of like the lifeguards at the swimming pool. Most of the time, all is well, but when you need them, you really need them. As a midwife, I'm always watching and observing, monitoring the "numbers" as well as subtler signs. Most of the time, that's all I do. However, there are those rare situations when I need to intervene quickly, efficiently, and without hesitation. This is why midwives spend years in training and participate in ongoing education. On those rare occasions when you need us to jump out of the lifeguard chair, we are well trained and fully equipped. This is midwifery, and all midwives take this responsibility seriously. At my birth center, for example, we have all the same first-line medications and equipment available in a hospital setting, and we're not shy about using them when necessary.

Additionally, we go through regular safety drills with our own staff, our emergency medical service partners, and our collaborating hospital.

If your labor becomes unexpectedly complicated, your midwife will not be mean to you and should not yell or become frazzled. However, they may not be able to have the thorough in-depth discussion you're used to having with them. In an emergency, things happen quickly, and the response must be equally rapid. The midwife should be able to swiftly tell you what's happening, so you know why your plans are being altered, but it's not the time for detailed explanations. Once you and your baby are stable and healthy, your midwife will be able to sit with you and have a comprehensive discussion about what happened and why.

Birth

Physically, there are many sensations happening all at once at the moment of birth. The contractions are powerful and strong, and the sensation of pressure in the rectum becomes even more intense. As the baby starts to crown (i.e., when the head is emerging), there will be a deep feeling of burning in your perineum, often referred to as the "ring of fire." The good news is that when you feel that ring of fire, it means you're at the finish line! Your midwife will be there to help support you and guide the baby out. Sometimes babies come out fast at the end, and your midwife may literally catch the baby! If your partner wants to catch the baby, the midwife will help them—and if you want to catch your baby, your midwife will help you with that as well.

Emotionally, the moment of birth is like no other that we experience. Labor may have been long and tiring and may have taken a different path than you planned, but none of that will matter when you feel the ecstasy and relief that accompany the powerful surge of hormones released as you give birth to your child. I have had laboring people and partners falling asleep in between contractions when pushing, laboring people who have given up and feel like the birth will never happen—all of these people have instantly lit up with joy and love when the birth happens. I call it "the human light bulb effect" because the mood in the room is so bright. Your midwife will help guard and create space for this moment to take place and unfold.

There will also be all kinds of fluids: mucus, amniotic fluid, sweat, and, of course, blood. But most of the time, there's not too much blood, and you'll be focused on your sweet baby as your birth team keeps track of the fluids, contains them, and cleans up the space. Soon after the birth, your midwife will gently wipe any excess fluids off the baby, except for the vernix, which is the thick, waxy, white substance that covers the baby's skin and essentially keeps them from becoming a little raisin in the amniotic fluid in the womb. It's best to let the vernix soak into the skin over the first hour or so because it helps keep the baby warm and acts as a moisturizer. At some point in the first 24 hours, you may wish to give the baby a bath, but it's very important to delay this for at least 8 to 12 hours, if not more. Newborns are highly susceptible to becoming dangerously cold, and bathing them too early can cause problems with their temperature.

The Third Stage of Labor

The third stage of labor is defined as the time from the birth of the baby until the expulsion of the placenta, or "afterbirth." The overall length of third stage can vary, but it typically lasts less than 30 minutes. This is a time when your midwife will be busy monitoring you and the baby to be sure you're both healthy and that your blood loss is within normal limits. Your midwife will also watch for signs of the placenta separating from the uterus as it prepares to be released. If you're giving birth in a community setting (at home or in a birth center), the midwife will typically have an assistant, either a registered nurse or someone with specific training as a birth assistant, to help them with all the necessary tasks. If you're in a hospital, there will be several other people in the room, some to help the midwife care for you and some to care for the baby. These details should be explained to you well before the birth so you know what to expect.

WHAT TO DO DURING THIRD STAGE

The third stage of labor is relatively short but can be very intense. You're processing the birth and focused on meeting this new little human you've created. This will be a time to catch your breath and soak in all the sensations and hormonal rushes. Some people need to take a moment to absorb all that's happened before they embrace the baby. Some people eagerly and immediately reach for their baby. There is no right or wrong way to be in this moment, and your midwife will support you in whichever way is appropriate for you.

At some point, as your placenta is getting close to delivery, you will feel a sensation of pressure—not as intense as when the baby came down but noticeable nonetheless. You might also feel cramping in your uterus. You may or may not need to bear down and give a small push, and your midwife may or may not need to apply some gentle traction on the umbilical cord as you push. Either way, your midwife will guide you to do what's most beneficial for your individual situation.

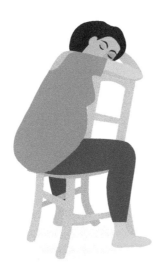

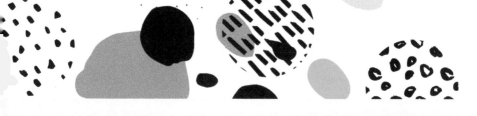

Birth Story: INVOLUTION INTERVENTION

Keisha was in labor with her third baby. Her first two births had been in a hospital, and though they hadn't been horrible, she and her husband, David, had opted for a more personalized experience in a freestanding birth center this time. Once she had birthed her beautiful baby into her husband's hands, we immediately placed the baby skin to skin on her abdomen, and David climbed in bed next to them.

I prepared for her third stage of labor and the delivery of the placenta. At first, the umbilical cord was thick and indigo in color, but over the course of a few minutes, as the baby received her blood, it became thinner and paler. Keisha reported some cramping, and the cord became longer as the placenta began to detach from the uterus. I applied gentle traction to the cord while asking her to give a little push. Her placenta slid out in one smooth motion. I then clamped the umbilical cord, and David cut it.

Keisha's first fundal massage revealed a firm, well-contracted uterus with minimal bleeding. But fifteen minutes later, during her next fundal massage, her uterus was soft, and she passed some large blood clots, followed by brisk, heavy bleeding. My nurse and I quickly did several things at once. I continued to vigorously massage her uterus as I ordered my nurse to inject medications into Keisha's thigh and start an IV line to give her fluids and more medication if needed. All the while, we were explaining everything to Keisha and her husband, and the baby remained blissfully cuddled on her chest. Within a

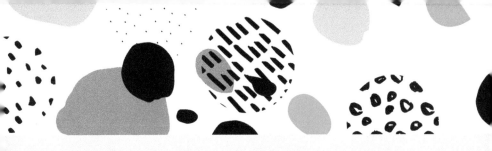

few minutes, the medications took effect, her uterus was once again firm, and her bleeding returned to normal. I ran fluids through her IV to help replace the volume she had lost due to the bleeding, and she didn't end up needing additional medication. Soon she felt much better, and she went home without any further complications.

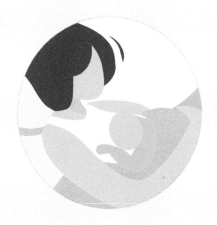

In the community setting, your midwife and their assistant will be responsible for the care of you and the baby. If you're in the hospital, your midwife will manage your care while nurses manage the care of the baby. In either setting, the midwife is responsible for ensuring that the placenta is birthed in a timely manner and that your bleeding is appropriate.

It's your midwife's job to manage all these issues so that you and your partner don't have to worry and can instead focus on the baby. Your partner and your doula will be focused on you and the baby in nonmedical ways, ensuring your comfort and helping support your emotional transition from labor to postpartum. Most of the time, all these things take place without too much interference in your bonding time as a new family.

If you're not keeping your placenta, it will be disposed of as biomedical waste. If you are keeping it (see page 80 for more information), various measures might be taken, depending on what you plan to do with it.

FUNDAL MASSAGE

Your uterus is not done working once you expel the placenta. In fact, it still has a very big job to do: It has to shrink back to its non-pregnant size, through a process called *involution*. This takes place over the following weeks, though it's at its most intense over the first hours and days after birth. Involution doesn't just help your uterus return to a more manageable size; it also prevents you from bleeding too much.

In the first few minutes after the placenta has been released, your midwife will need to assess that the process is taking place properly by performing something called "fundal massage." Even though this process has the word "massage" in it, it's usually not pleasant. Your midwife will rub your abdomen in the area above your pubic bone and below your belly button to make sure that involution is happening, your uterus is firm, and you're not losing an excessive amount of blood. It's something your midwife (or their assistant or nurse) needs to do for your safety, even though it's not enjoyable.

This fundal massage is usually done several times in the first hour and then less frequently as the hours progress. You may experience menstrual-like cramps in between fundal massages as the uterus continues involuting on its own. If your uterus isn't firm or you're bleeding heavily, the massage may be more vigorous and occur more frequently. In some cases, your midwife may need to give you medication to help the uterus involute more quickly. If you're in a hospital, your nurse will likely do the actual massage and then notify your midwife if there are any concerns.

POTENTIAL COMPLICATIONS IN THIRD STAGE

Third-stage potential problems primarily have to do with the placenta and your bleeding. These can include retained placenta (when the placenta doesn't deliver after an appropriate time) and postpartum hemorrhage (more blood loss than expected). In healthy births, these are rare; however, if they do occur, they can happen very quickly, and your midwife may need to make fast decisions and act very rapidly. If you're in the hospital, they may call for more personnel to come to the room as well as a physician. If you're in the community setting, they may need to activate their emergency transport plans. In either setting, the midwife may need to administer medications to help control the situation.

Immediately after Birth

After the third stage of labor and birth, once your placenta has been safely delivered, the real work of bonding and recovery begins. Your midwife and their assistant/nurse will take care of the details and clean up so you don't have to worry. Your baby will be placed skin to skin on your abdomen or chest. This is one of the most profound moments in a person's life and should be cherished. If both mother and baby are well, your midwife will help safeguard this time and make sure it's not interrupted. Your midwife will make sure the baby is breathing properly and is being kept warm, and your partner will be there to assist you and offer support.

CORD CLAMPING

The umbilical cord is what connects the baby to the placenta, delivering nutrients, getting rid of waste, and so on. Now that the baby is born, they no longer need it, so at some point, the umbilical cord will need to be clamped and then cut.

The cord can be cut by the co-parent, the birthing parent, another family member, your midwife, or anyone you choose. For some families, it's an important ritual-like event, and for others it's not. Either way is correct, as long as it's what you decide. Your midwife will assist the person cutting the cord by helping position the baby, preparing the cord, and instructing them in how to cut it. Umbilical cords are tough and thick, so it can take some gentle force to cut all the way through. The baby won't feel it, as there are no nerve endings in the cord, but they might fuss a bit about the process. Keeping them skin to skin will help comfort them.

The timing of the cutting and clamping of the umbilical cord can have lasting effects for your newborn. Many hospitals and providers clamp the cord within seconds of birth, which is known as "immediate" (or "premature") cord clamping. Many midwives, on the other hand, practice "physiologic" or "delayed" cord clamping, which can take up to five or ten minutes (or even longer).

What's the thinking behind delayed cord clamping? At birth, your newborn has roughly 85 milliliters of blood for every two pounds of their weight. For reference, this means that if your baby weighs seven pounds, they have a little over one cup of blood. For the last few months of your pregnancy, this volume of blood has been circulating through the baby, the umbilical cord, and the fetal side of the placenta—but it all belongs to the baby. It's the volume the baby's body is accustomed to functioning with. Immediately after birth, approximately 80 to 100 milliliters of that blood is still in the umbilical cord. This may not seem like a lot, but for your baby, it can represent up to one-quarter to one-third of their total blood volume. If you suddenly lost that much blood, you'd feel it! By waiting a few minutes to cut the cord, you allow the blood from the umbilical cord to flow into the baby. That's the point of physiologic cord clamping: It lets your baby keep all their own blood.

Delayed cord clamping results in many short- and long-term benefits for your baby. These include increased oxygenation in the baby's brain, increased iron reserves for the first six months, increased myelination (improved nervous system and brain development), and a decreased chance of needing blood or iron transfusions. There is even some data that suggests that babies who experience physiologic cord clamping have improved fine motor and social skills years later. There is also some evidence that suggests a slightly higher rate of jaundice (yellowing of the skin) in newborns after physiologic cord clamping, but the benefits outweigh this risk.

SKIN-TO-SKIN CONTACT

The baby should be kept skin to skin for the first few hours after birth, on either the birthing parent or the co-parent. (Skin-to-skin time counts for both parents!) In fact, I encourage skin-to-skin contact—with either parent—for the first 72 hours. It has been proven to have multiple health benefits for the birthing parent, the baby, and even the co-parent. These include improved rates of breast/chest feeding, less overall blood loss for the mother, improved satisfaction with the birth, and an increased sense of bonding. Babies who experience skin-to-skin care have better self-regulation of temperature, heart rate, and breathing patterns. For the co-parent, this practice also enhances bonding and attachment. Your midwife will be instrumental in ensuring that this skin-to-skin contact happens immediately and will educate you on continuing it beyond the first few hours.

BREAST/CHEST FEEDING

Another top priority immediately after birth should be breast/chest feeding. (If you cannot or have decided not to do so for whatever reason, then you'll feed the baby with a bottle during this time.) Breast/chest feeding is a process that sometimes happens easily and quickly and can sometimes be more challenging. Either way, you're not alone. You will have prepared for this by taking classes during your pregnancy, and your midwife, partner, and any other members of your birth team will be there to support and guide you.

POTENTIAL COMPLICATIONS IMMEDIATELY AFTER GIVING BIRTH

For most low-risk, healthy people, the immediate postpartum period will be smooth and gentle, focused on the baby, bonding, and feeding. But there are some rare complications that can happen immediately after third stage. It's uncommon in healthy, full-term newborns, but the baby could need extra help breathing. If this rare emergency happens in the hospital, your baby may be transferred to the neonatal intensive care unit (NICU). If you have not given birth at a hospital, your midwife will activate their emergency transport plans and have the baby taken to the NICU. In either case, you'll be temporarily separated from the baby, but in many cases, the co-parent can accompany the baby until you can join them.

During the immediate postpartum period, your midwife will need to closely examine your vagina and perineum for any lacerations that may have occurred. They will do this with your permission and will talk you through the process, informing you of what they're doing and seeing. The initial exam can feel uncomfortable, as they will need to see the tissue, which requires some manipulation. If a laceration is discovered, your midwife will discuss it with you, and together you can decide if you'll get stitches to repair it. Not all lacerations require stitches, but many do. Please know that if you do require a repair, your midwife should offer to administer local anesthesia prior to suturing. Laceration repairs are typically done within the first hour, but your midwife may delay them slightly, depending on the whole picture of your recovery. The vast majority of lacerations will be relatively minor to moderate, and your midwife will be able to repair them. In the rare case of a severe laceration, a physician will be called in (if you're in a hospital), or your midwife will activate their transport plans to take you to the hospital.

The First 24 Hours

The first 24 hours after delivering your baby will likely fly by! So much happens during this time that it can seem unreal. You'll be focused on bonding with and feeding your baby as well as on the work of physical recovery. Even though birth is a well-designed process, it's also a massive undertaking that requires time and support to heal from. These first hours are all about resting, eating and drinking, keeping baby skin to skin (on either parent), and . . . going to the bathroom.

Yes, getting up to use the restroom is very important. In order for your uterus to complete the process of involution, your bladder must be emptied frequently. If it's not, you're more likely to have significant bleeding, which can lead to a postpartum hemorrhage. When you get up to go to the bathroom, you will also be able to perform "peri care," which means keeping your perineal area clean and managing healing if you had a laceration with or without stitches. Typically, this includes using a squirt bottle (called a "peri bottle") filled with warm water to clean the area after peeing, taking a warm Epsom salt bath, and applying topical comfort remedies such as arnica oil, cold packs, witch hazel, and/or aloe. Your midwife will guide you to the interventions that best fit your individual situation.

Where you gave birth will have a large impact on this first day, but no matter the setting, you will not be without support in these first 24 hours. Here's how it looks in the various locations.

THE FIRST 24 HOURS AFTER A HOME BIRTH

If you give birth at home, your midwife and their assistant will remain at your home for between two and six hours, though the length may depend on your individual midwife. They'll be sure that you and your baby are healthy and well, assist with breast/chest feeding, and do some cleanup of the space. When they do leave, they'll give you instructions for your aftercare and encourage you to contact them with any questions or concerns.

One benefit of giving birth at home is that you'll be in your own space, with your own clothes and comfort items. You'll be able to use your own bathroom for peeing, performing your peri care, and taking Epsom salt baths. Your kitchen and preferred foods will be easily available. It is also very easy for your support team to assist you.

THE FIRST 24 HOURS AFTER BIRTH AT A BIRTH CENTER

If you give birth in a freestanding birth center with your midwife, you'll complete the immediate recovery at the center. Typically, families remain at the center for a period of 4 to 12 hours after the birth, though each center has its own guidelines. During this time, your midwife and their assistant will be present to help with all the aftercare. They will make sure that you and the baby are well, help you feed the baby, assist you to the bathroom, and teach you about peri care. In most centers, they'll prepare food for you and your partner to eat. At my center, we prepare a warm Epsom salt bath for our postpartum people to enjoy before going home. Your midwife or their assistant will go over all of your discharge instructions and help you to your car. Once home, you'll be able to recover in your own space as with a home birth.

THE FIRST 24 HOURS AFTER A HOSPITAL BIRTH

If you have decided on a hospital birth with your midwife, you'll likely remain at the hospital for 24 to 48 hours. Your midwife will be with you for the first hour or so postpartum, and then the nursing staff will oversee your care. In some hospitals, you'll be moved to a new room, and in others you'll stay in the same room you gave birth in. Your nurse will make sure you and your baby are healthy, help you feed the baby, and contact your midwife for instructions if they have any concerns.

Your nurse will also help you go to the bathroom. (If you had an epidural, you'll need to wait for it to wear off before you can get out of bed and walk.) In terms of peri care, most hospitals don't have full-size bathtubs for Epsom salt baths, but they may have a small basin that fits over the toilet to let you have a sitz bath, which soaks your perineum only. Depending on the specific hospital and time you give birth, if the cafeteria is closed, you may not be able to order a full meal right away, but most units have some snacks and pre-packaged items like sandwiches. Your midwife will visit you the next day to check in on you and the day after that to help you get discharged home.

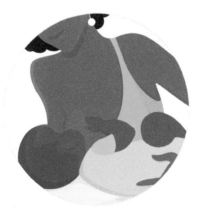

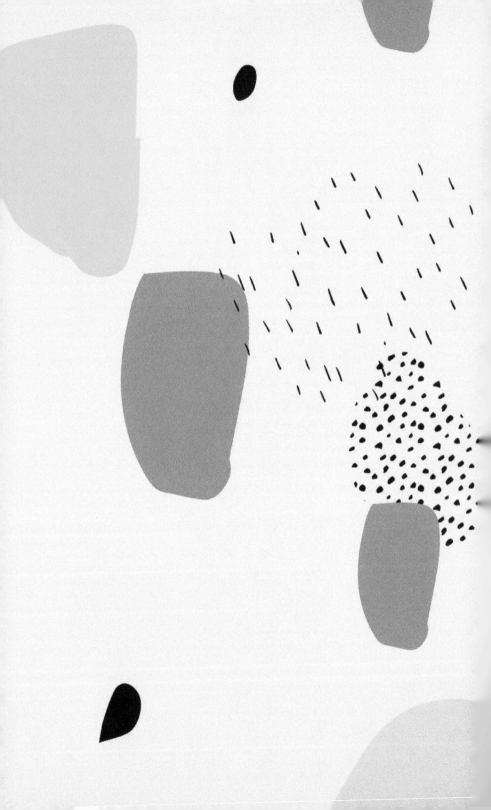

CHAPTER 6

Midwifery after Birth

Once your baby is born, the work is not over. It's kind of like the relationship between a wedding and a marriage. The wedding is important, but it's only one day—the ensuing marriage is really what it's all about. Pregnancy and birth are the preparation for the real transformation of becoming a parent and the ongoing task of parenting. Once you give birth, your midwife does not disappear. In fact, you may rely more on your midwife to guide you through these first intense, tumultuous, and beautiful weeks.

Postpartum Midwifery

The initial postpartum period can feel like a blur. There are sleepless nights, dirty diapers, milk-stained clothes, and spit-up everywhere. It's also full of wonderful moments: the way the baby fits in your arms, snuggly early mornings, and sunshiny smiles. It is simultaneously exhausting and exhilarating. Much like parenting overall, it is the best thing and the hardest thing. There will be amazingly wonderful days, days when you'll feel broken, and all the possibilities in between. Having the support of your family, friends, midwife, lactation specialists, and potentially a postpartum doula can help alleviate some the weight as you adjust to this new reality.

Your midwife's job is not finished with the birth of your baby. They'll continue to walk with you on this journey through the first few weeks, offering emotional support as well as monitoring your physical safety and recovery. Here are a few of the things you can expect from your midwife immediately postpartum:

- Checking in on your mental health status to monitor for postpartum depression

- Making sure any perineal lacerations are healing properly

- Going over the signs of mastitis (an infection that can happen in the breasts) and treating it if it does happen

- Making sure your postpartum bleeding is within normal limits

- Answering any questions about feeding, well-baby care, and the normal course of healing for your body

You'll have built a relationship with your midwife over the course of your pregnancy. You can turn to them for knowledge, and they'll be there to answer your questions. Additionally, midwives are generally excellent at connecting folks with other providers and specialists. They will likely know all the lactation consultants, pelvic-floor physical therapists, baby-wearing experts, and postpartum doulas in your area.

POSTPARTUM DOULAS

Like labor/birth doulas and sibling doulas, postpartum doulas are another specialty in the doula world. They're trained to provide support and education to new parents and will do so in your home. They can be there during the day or at night, performing light household duties and helping you learn baby care and breast/chest feeding. Each postpartum doula will offer specific services and have individual skill sets. As with a birth doula, you can interview several to find the one that best fits your family.

Postpartum Checkups with a Midwife

The type, frequency, and location of postpartum visits will depend on both your midwife and your birth setting. Midwives who work in the community setting (in the home or in a birth center) will likely offer several postpartum face-to-face visits. For example, in my practice as a birth-center midwife, our clients receive a phone call approximately 24 hours after the birth, a comprehensive exam of both the postpartum person and the newborn 2 days after the birth, and another of these "double" exam visits 8 to 10 days after the birth. At these visits, we do all the same screening and testing for the newborn that would be done at a hospital or pediatrician's office. If we feel we need to see a family more—for, say, feeding support or emotional support—we will. Then we see the postpartum person at six weeks after the birth. Home-birth midwives offer a similar schedule, with the possibility of even more visits.

Where will your postpartum visits take place? If you gave birth at a birth center, these visits typically take place in the center's clinic, though some birth centers offer one home visit in the first few days after birth. Home-birth midwives usually conduct their visits in your home. Midwives who work in the hospital setting may not physically see their clients until the six-week visit but will be available to offer support and guidance over the phone when necessary and can always bring you into their offices if there are any concerns. Regardless of the type of midwife, if your postpartum recovery is normal, you won't need to see a physician during this time. Your midwife is well trained to provide all of this care.

POSTPARTUM CHECKUPS
FOR YOUR NEWBORN

It's important to have an in-depth conversation with your midwife about how much and what type of newborn care they offer. Many hospital-based midwives don't offer any newborn care and will immediately refer you to a pediatrician (whom you'll have interviewed and chosen during your pregnancy). Community midwives often offer extensive newborn care such as weight monitoring, jaundice assessment and treatment, and routine screenings like hearing tests. Certified nurse midwives (CNMs), for example, are trained and certified to provide well-baby care for the first month of life. At my birth center, if a newborn has a normal course, we discharge them from our care after the 8- to 10-day exam, and our families schedule an appointment with a pediatrician for the 14-day exam. If your baby needs pediatric care sooner, your midwife will refer you sooner.

POSTPARTUM CHECKUPS FOR YOU

The physical exam at a postpartum checkup will involve things like listening to your heart and lungs, taking your blood pressure, assessing your breasts and nipples (with your consent), examining your uterus to make sure it's involuting, and checking in on your bleeding. On at least one of these visits, your midwife will probably ask permission to look at your perineum and vagina, particularly if you had a laceration, to make sure everything is healing well and there are no signs of infection. Depending on your health history and how your birth went, they may also draw blood to check for problems, like anemia after a postpartum hemorrhage.

Your postpartum visits won't just be about your physical health—your midwife will want to check in on your mental health as well. They will likely screen for postpartum depression and ask you questions like: How is newborn feeding going? What is your bleeding like? Do you have any pain in your perineum or vagina? Do you have any questions about your birth?

At the final six-week postpartum exam, your midwife may perform all the examinations listed previously and then ask permission to conduct an internal pelvic exam. This exam will check your pelvic-floor muscle strength and make sure that any lacerations have healed. If your midwife has concerns, they may recommend home exercises or a pelvic-floor physical therapist. They'll also assess your abdominal muscles, which can sometimes separate during pregnancy in a way that's difficult to fully heal from. (If this is the case, your midwife will discuss and recommend a physical therapist.)

Finally, a big component of the final visit is to discuss family planning and contraception plans. Midwives are well versed in all available types of contraception, from barrier methods to natural family planning to birth control pills to intrauterine devices (IUDs). They will help you choose a method that works best for you and your lifestyle.

Bonding with Baby

Some parents feel an instant bond with their baby, while others may need time to build that bond. Either situation is normal, so don't judge yourself harshly if you fall into the latter group. One critical step for bonding with your baby is time spent skin to skin, particularly immediately after birth and for the first 72 hours. (See "Skin-to-Skin Contact" on page 120 for more details.)

As the days progress and you spend more time with the baby, in most cases, the bond will continue to form and strengthen. Again, if you don't feel some magical instant connection, that's okay. For some parents, it takes days, weeks, or even months to build that bond. As long as you feel able to care for the baby—feed them, hold them, change their diapers, bathe them—the best thing to do is continue with those tasks. The bond will eventually form.

If at any point you don't feel like you're able to do these tasks in a positive way, reach out to your support team. Talk to your partner and call your midwife right away. These can be signs of significant postpartum depression and should be assessed immediately. (See page 137 for more details.) Help is available, and your midwife can guide you to the support and intervention that you and your family need. If you experience postpartum depression, please remember that it is not your fault and it does not mean that you're a bad parent. It simply means that you may need more intensive support to move past this phase.

Postpartum Self-Care

In the first few weeks, it's all too easy to be so focused on the new baby that you forget to care for yourself. But in order to best care for your baby, *you* need to be cared for, too. Self-care is not selfish—it is vital to being a good caregiver.

GET SOME REST

As we have discussed, giving birth is hard work. This massive transformation takes vast reserves of energy. During this recovery phase, you need time and support to heal yourself while also learning how to parent.

One of the best things you can do for yourself in the first two weeks after birth is rest. Stay at home and cocoon yourself. Give yourself space to sleep when you can, snuggle with the baby, and just be. Rest, rest, rest, and then rest some more. This may sound silly, but I'm very serious. If you can get two weeks of recuperation and quiet space at home, your overall recovery will be supported and shortened. I know this can be difficult, but please believe me when I say it: Resting will pay off in the long run.

This isn't to say that you should be bedridden, but I recommend trying to remain in your own space. The birthing parent should not be out running errands, cleaning the house, hosting guests and visitors, or preparing all the meals. This is a time to use your community. Our current mainstream culture puts a high value on the concept of independence, but in the postpartum recovery period, we need our communities. Humans are social animals who thrive in groups. Traditionally, when a family had just welcomed a new baby, folks helped with cooking, housework, and yardwork without expecting to be entertained. We need to reclaim this time and phase in our lives by allowing this help. When someone asks you what they can do to help, don't just brush them off. Take them up on their offer—you may be surprised at how happy it makes them to help and be involved.

Starting in the third week and beyond, it can be time to start taking short, easy walks in the sun. Nothing too hard or demanding—just a simple stroll. Over the next few weeks, you can build up the walking time and length. Enjoy being outside, get some fresh air, and breathe in the oxygen. Feel your muscles waking and warming up. Pay attention to your bleeding; if it increases after being active, that's a signal you may have been too active and need to back down a little.

During this recovery period, your midwife is an invaluable resource and will support you and guide you back to feeling like yourself. Part of that six-week postpartum check is to be sure you're ready to get back to your pre-pregnancy lifestyle. You can always come to your midwife with questions about rest and other forms of caring for your physical health.

TAKING CARE OF YOUR MIND

Becoming a parent is a powerful, all-encompassing transformation—all while you're also trying to learn how to care for a small baby who is completely dependent on you for survival. (No pressure!) Most people—up to 80 percent—will experience something colloquially referred to as the "baby blues." This is different from postpartum depression and usually occurs in the first two weeks after birth as your hormonal systems are returning to a pre-pregnancy baseline.

These two weeks can feel a bit like an emotional roller coaster. You might be happy and laughing one moment and then crying the next. This is usually very normal. Let yourself feel what you need to feel. If you have any questions or trauma around your birth, talk about it with your partner, your midwife, and maybe even a therapist. Don't bottle things up—let them all flow out. For most people, as you come out of that two-week haze, your emotions will begin to feel more normal.

One of the most important components of mental and emotional self-care is getting adequate sleep. We often make jokes about how exhausted new parents are, but sleep deprivation is real. Work with your community (partner, family, midwife, postpartum doula) to create a sleep plan. This may sound like overkill, but it's not. You need sleep! Make it a priority, schedule it, make sure it happens. You likely won't be able to get a full eight hours of sleep, especially if you're breast/chest feeding, but you can typically figure out a way to get three or four hours, which will feel like a miracle.

And don't forget your partner! They should have a sleep plan, too. They will also be tired and going through the transformation of becoming a new parent. If they're also deeply sleep deprived, they won't be able to give you the best support.

Make sure not to isolate yourself. After those first two weeks of cocooning at home, get out for small trips. Engage with the community by attending groups for new parents, going to lactation support groups, and visiting with your friends and family. Your midwife will be able to guide you toward these resources in your community. There is power in being with other families who are going through the same things you are. It's comforting to know you're not alone.

Finally, the gentle return to physical activity detailed previously is healthy for your mind as well as your body. This triad of adequate sleep, avoiding isolation, and gentle exercise is crucial for improving and supporting your postpartum mental health.

POSTPARTUM DEPRESSION

Postpartum depression (PPD) is different from the baby blues and can affect up to 15 percent of postpartum people. The term "postpartum depression" can be misleading; some people experience PPD more as anxiety than as sadness. PPD can happen to any person regardless of age, number of babies, support level, ethnicity, or financial situation. If you have a personal or family history of depression, mental health concerns, or substance use disorder, the risk of developing PPD can be higher. If you experience PPD, the most important thing to remember is that **it is not your fault and it does not mean you don't love your baby**. It also **does not make you a bad parent**. It just means that you'll require extra care and support.

Your midwife will be instrumental in screening for PPD. During the pregnancy, if they identify any risk factors, they'll discuss those with you and make a plan to monitor for the symptoms. During the postpartum period, they will screen both formally and informally for any potential symptoms and new risk factors.

If your midwife diagnoses you with PPD, they'll consult with mental health providers in your area to create a treatment plan. PPD can be treated and is not usually a permanent diagnosis, but it can last up to or past the first 12 to 24 months. The first-line treatment should be counseling, either in a one-on-one setting with a therapist or in a group facilitated by a therapist. For many people, therapy coupled with support at home, regular sleep, and moderate exercise will help alleviate the symptoms. Some people require all of these interventions as well as prescription medication. Depending on the type of midwife you have, they may be able to prescribe this medication. If they can't, they'll direct you to community resources who can.

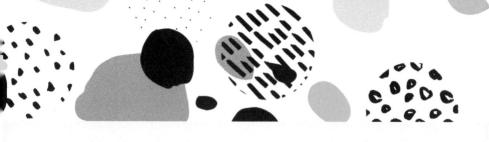

Birth Story: OVERCOMING PPD

Monica had recently given birth to her third child. It was a normal pregnancy and birth without any major issues. But during her postpartum visits, the midwifery team noticed that Monica seemed withdrawn, her usual bubbly personality muted. She was tired and unenthusiastic about the baby, overly worried, and on edge. Four weeks after the birth, we diagnosed her with PPD. With the support of her family, we immediately made lifestyle adjustment plans: scheduling sleep, getting regular exercise, and receiving help with household chores. Next, we connected her with a therapist for counseling. For a few weeks, these interventions seemed to have a positive impact. But at a follow-up appointment with me a few weeks later, it became clear that they were no longer offering enough help.

Monica and I had a long conversation about how she was feeling. Her therapist had also been concerned that she was losing ground. Together, we decided that Monica would continue with therapy and lifestyle interventions, *and* we would also add in a prescription antidepressant. I thoroughly reviewed her health history and, taking into account that she was still exclusively breastfeeding, decided on a particular medication. She started it the next day.

Over the next few months, Monica began to make steady progress back toward her pre-PPD mental health. She had frequent appointments with me to monitor the medication and continued to see her therapist. Shortly after her baby's first

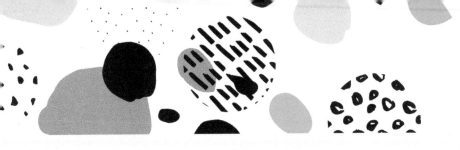

birthday, we decided to see if she could wean off the prescription. This was done gradually, with lots of follow-up over the phone and in person. Eventually, she was able to completely come off the medication. Monica continued to see her therapist, though with less frequency, and returned to a mental state that was normal for her. Today, years later, she is a strong, thriving mother and human.

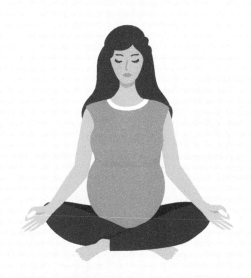

Infant Feeding

Choosing how you'll feed your baby is an important decision. Whether you choose formula or human milk, be informed and feel confident in your choice. Your midwife can help review the options with you.

Many people will opt to breast/chest feed their baby, especially in the beginning. There are several evidence-based reasons to choose this option—it offers many health benefits for the baby and for the lactating parent, too. For the baby, breast milk provides the most nutritionally appropriate food available. It's full of immune-system boosters, and it changes with your baby, adjusting to their nutritional needs as they develop and grow. It also helps protect against sudden infant death syndrome (SIDS), some infections, diarrhea, type 2 diabetes, and childhood obesity. For the lactating parent, nursing helps decrease your postpartum bleeding, encourages bonding, and can even help prevent breast and ovarian cancer as well as autoimmune diseases later in life. For all these reasons and more, breast/chest feeding is considered the optimal choice.

However, it may not be the right choice for you, depending on your specific situation. All people should be supported in making the best choice for themselves and their baby. Some people are not able to breast/chest feed for personal reasons. For example, survivors of sexual assault or abuse may find it retraumatizing. Others can't breastfeed due to physical conditions, like a history of breast surgery. (These surgeries don't always prevent nursing. If you've had one, discuss it with your midwife.)

If you can't or don't want to breast/chest feed, there are other options, such as using formula or human milk donated through a milk bank. If this is the route you take, there is no need to feel guilty or like you've failed. Feeding the baby is always the right choice, and your midwife can help support you through any potential negative feelings this can cause.

No matter how you decide to feed your baby, your midwife will be involved in supporting you. Midwives receive training in lactation and infant feeding and have good knowledge about ways to help you succeed. Many doulas also have additional training in this area, and lactation consultants are experts on it. Your midwife can likely refer you to lactation consultants they know and trust.

Breast/Chest Feeding Problems and How to Fix Them

As with any other natural biological process, sometimes complications can arise when breast/chest feeding. Occasionally, some people find they can't produce enough milk, in which case a midwife and/or lactation consultant can offer many tried-and-true interventions to increase your supply. Breast size alone is not an indicator of milk production (small-breasted people can usually produce plenty of milk), but nipple size and shape can affect your ability to nurse. Having flat or inverted nipples doesn't automatically mean you won't be able to breastfeed, but you may need extra support, including a tool called a nipple shield to assist with latching. During your pregnancy, your midwife will do an assessment of your breasts and nipples to identify any potential concerns and formulate a plan to deal with them if needed.

Let's take a closer look at some common breast/chest feeding problems and how to solve them.

ENGORGEMENT

Engorgement may happen in the first few days postpartum as your milk comes in if your baby is not able to empty your breasts well.

Symptoms

Breasts will be uncomfortably large, hard, and possibly reddened. (Don't be worried that this "should" happen. If you don't experience this, that's good!) Due to the firmness, it may be difficult to latch the baby.

Remedies

Try using an electric or manual breast pump for a few minutes. Or you can stand in a warm shower to help loosen the breasts and then hand express (squeeze the milk out with your hand) to relieve some of the pressure. Try to express just enough milk to get the breasts softer so the baby can latch.

CLOGGED MILK DUCTS

Clogged ducts occur anytime milk gets "stuck" or backed up in a milk duct. It's important to take care of them quickly because if left untreated, they can develop into mastitis.

Symptoms

A hard lump in one or both breasts that may also be warm to the touch and reddened. The lump might be the size of a pea, a grape, or even a small lime.

Remedies

Prepare a warm castor oil compress by gently heating castor oil in a double boiler on the stovetop and soaking a clean washcloth in the oil. Wrap the cloth around the affected area and then wrap the washcloth with plastic wrap so the heat stays on the breast instead of dissipating into the air. Leave it in place for 10 to 15 minutes; then completely wipe the oil off your breast and either use a breast pump or latch the baby to that breast. As you do so, also apply vibration to the clogged spot using the non-bristle end of an electric toothbrush. This will usually break up the clog, though you may need to repeat the process several times.

If you're prone to clogs, I recommend a daily preventive supplement called lecithin that can be found in any health-food store.

MASTITIS

Mastitis is a very serious infection in the breast tissue. Note that the infection is *not* present in the milk itself, and if you have mastitis, you must keep emptying the breasts by nursing the baby, hand expressing, or using a pump.

Symptoms
Mastitis has flu-like symptoms that come on fast and intense, including a fever, body aches, and chills.

Remedies
Once you have mastitis, the recommended remedy is oral antibiotics. If your midwife can't prescribe them, they'll consult with someone who can. Be sure to take the full course of the medication even if you start to feel better.

THRUSH

Thrush is a fungal infection by a type of naturally occurring yeast called candida—it's essentially a yeast infection but in your nipples and/or your baby's mouth. Yes, it can be passed from parent to child and vice versa, so you might have to treat both yourself and your baby.

Symptoms

Thrush symptoms for you: reddened, flaky nipples and sharp stabbing pain that radiates from the nipples deep into the breast. These symptoms can affect one or both breasts.

Thrush symptoms for your child: white patches on the inside of their cheeks and/or a red, blotchy diaper rash.

Remedies

Everything that comes into contact with your nipples can have candida yeast living on it, so you must meticulously clean and sterilize all your bras, reusable nursing pads, breast-pump supplies, and baby bottles and nipples. You can also apply a topical solution of a compound called gentian violet (less than 0.5 percent concentration) to the nipples after nursing for a period of no more than 7 days. (Be careful—it will permanently stain any cloth it touches a dark purple!) If these interventions don't work, your midwife can prescribe a medication called nystatin that can treat both you and the baby.

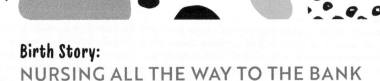

Birth Story:
NURSING ALL THE WAY TO THE BANK

Jasmine and her partner had just welcomed their first baby. The labor had been long, and after the birth, she experienced a postpartum hemorrhage. We were able to stop the bleeding at the birth center, but she lost enough blood that we decided to transport her and the baby to the hospital. After 36 hours, Jasmine's blood tests were normal, she felt better, and she went home.

Typically, it can take 36 to 48 hours after birth for the full milk to come in. It's a massive metabolic demand on your body, and any deviations from normalcy during or after the birth—such as a postpartum hemorrhage—can cause delays. This was the case for Jasmine. After 48 hours, her milk still hadn't come in. The baby was fussy and hungry, and Jasmine was exhausted and frustrated.

Luckily, we were able to give them extra midwifery support, bring in a lactation consultant, and supply them with donor milk. My community is blessed to have a public human-milk bank that accepts donated breast milk from highly screened community members and processes it for use by babies who need it. Sometimes these are sick babies in the hospital; other times, they're well babies who just need supplementation for a day or two. Jasmine and her baby only needed the donated milk for two days. On day four, her milk came in. In the end, this precious resource let her meet her personal goal of breastfeeding her baby for one full year.

Caring for Your Newborn

Caring for your newborn can feel like a monumental task, but your midwife and the rest of your support team will be there to help guide you through the process for the first six weeks. Midwives have training and education on caring for healthy newborns and will be a great source of information that you can continue to build on long after you and your midwife part ways. However, one discussion that is best had with your pediatrician rather than your midwife is related to vaccinations. Your midwife may have some resources on this, but it's your pediatrician who will be caring for your baby in the long run, and they should be your primary go-to when making these decisions.

As you read about some of the basics of newborn care, remember that you're the one with the final say in all these decisions. Being a parent means constantly making choices about everything, and you'll probably be receiving conflicting advice from care providers, friends, family, and even random people off the street. This can feel overwhelming and confusing. But at the end of the day, you're the one who needs to decide how you want to parent. I always tell families that none of these people offering advice will be there with you at 2:00 in the morning when it counts. That will be up to you and your partner, so do what works best for your family.

DIAPERING

During the first few weeks, you might be shocked by how all-consuming the task of changing diapers becomes. You'll spend time analyzing the contents of your baby's diaper and find yourself having full-fledged conversations with other people about them! Don't worry—all parents have been there, and it won't last forever. In the first few days, you'll need to pay attention to the diaper count, as this will let you be sure the baby is getting enough food. What goes in must come out, and if they're making urine and stool, it means they're eating well.

The first stool, called "meconium," is passed during those first few days. It is odorless, thick, and sticky, with the consistency of brownie batter. If it dries before you can change the diaper, it will stick to the baby's skin and can be difficult to remove. To avoid this, I recommend that parents place a tiny amount of olive oil on and around the anus and buttocks after changing a diaper so that the next round of meconium doesn't stick to the skin. If it does dry on, place a washcloth with warm water over the area to rewet the poop before trying to remove it.

When changing a baby girl's diapers, always clean from the front to the back—you don't want to wipe poop up toward the vulva, as this can lead to infections. Also, don't significantly open the labia and wipe in the vagina, as doing so can cause irritation. Some baby girls may have a mini menstrual period as they're withdrawing from the maternal hormones. It won't be heavy bleeding, just a couple of drops. This is very normal, but you can always call your midwife or pediatrician for reassurance.

When changing a baby boy's diapers, be sure to lift the testicles as poop can "hide" under them. When closing the diaper after changing it, be sure to point the penis down. Otherwise, when he pees, it will shoot up and out of the diaper. Note that it's very normal for baby boys to have erections when you open the diaper and the cool air hits the penis. Be careful—when that happens, the pee can go anywhere!

BATHING

As mentioned earlier, it's important to delay the first bath until 8 to 12 hours after birth at least, since baths any sooner than that can dangerously lower a baby's body temperature. After that initial bath, you'll need to wait until the umbilical cord stump falls off to give your baby a full-body bath, as you don't want the stump to get too wet. Once the stump has fallen off, you can start giving more regular baths, but be careful. Typically, two to three baths per week is enough—if you bathe your baby too often, it can lead to skin irritation. Just be sure to keep the diaper area clean in between full baths.

Bathing a baby in the first days and weeks can be very intimidating! Once you get your baby wet, they become pretty slippery, so you'll want to get all your supplies handy ahead of time: body wash, shampoo, washcloths, dry towels, a fresh diaper (or two), and clothes to dress the baby in. No matter what, you cannot leave the baby in the bath to go and get anything you don't have right there. If you do forget something, have another person bring it to you, or take the baby out of the tub and take them with you to retrieve what you forgot. Be sure the ambient room temperature is nice and warm, and test whether the water is too hot by running it over the soft skin of your inner wrist.

WHERE WILL BABY SLEEP?

When it comes to where your baby will sleep, you'll be bombarded with opinions from all sides. Some will tell you adamantly never to sleep with your baby, while others will say just as adamantly never to put them in a crib. You can develop your own plan based on these facts, drawn from American Academy of Pediatrics (AAP) guidelines:

- Place your baby on their back on a firm surface to sleep.

- Be sure there are no excess pillows, blankets, toys, or objects that the baby could become tangled in. This includes products sold as "sleep positioners," as they can interfere with your baby's breathing. (If the baby is sleeping with you, each parent can have a pillow, but they should be kept clear of the baby.)

- Keep the ambient room temperature warm so the baby doesn't have to be overly swaddled or covered. Typically, babies only require one more layer of clothing than you're wearing.

- Never sleep in a chair, recliner, or couch with your baby. It's too easy for the baby to become wedged between you and the cushions and suffocate. If you're holding your baby in a recliner or couch and are becoming tired, get up and put the baby in a safe place.

The AAP also recommends that your baby sleep in a bassinet in your room for the first six months but cautions against co-sleeping or bed-sharing with your baby. Other experts and organizations such as La Leche League recommend co-sleeping for exclusively breastfed infants. In addition to the preceding recommendations, these groups also recommend the parents be sober and non-smokers. Ultimately, you'll need to make the choice that best fits you and your family.

Farewell to the Midwife

Once you've navigated the wild ride of pregnancy, birth, and the initial six postpartum weeks, your relationship with your birth team will change. If you worked with a doula, their services will end (unless you're working with a postpartum doula and extend their services beyond six weeks). For most healthy folks, that six-week postpartum exam will be the last one, and you'll officially be discharged from your midwife's care for this pregnancy. The baby will start seeing their pediatrician either immediately after the birth or in the first few days or weeks, and then regularly over the first year. You won't need to see another provider or physician.

This can be a bittersweet time for everyone, including your midwife. Pregnancy and especially birth are very intimate events that often lead to a strong bond between those who share it with each other. It's easy for the midwife to feel like part of your family, and saying goodbye can be difficult.

The good news is that it doesn't have to be a forever farewell. You may decide that your family is not complete and return to your midwife for subsequent births. I have several families for whom I've attended the births of multiple children. Plus, as I've mentioned, many midwives also provide comprehensive and full-scope women's health care. I love to see all my clients back around the baby's first birthday for their annual well-woman exam. And many of my clients keep me on as a primary care provider, since I'm a certified nurse midwife and can offer those services.

Sharing my knowledge and experience throughout the pages of this book has been a great honor and privilege for me. For me, being a midwife is both a calling and a profession. Being invited into your life through these pages has allowed me to embrace this work more fully and to support more families than I ever could in person. My deepest wish is that you have found it to be helpful and informative. I hope you feel empowered and prepared to tackle this amazing journey.

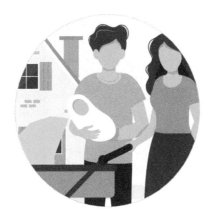

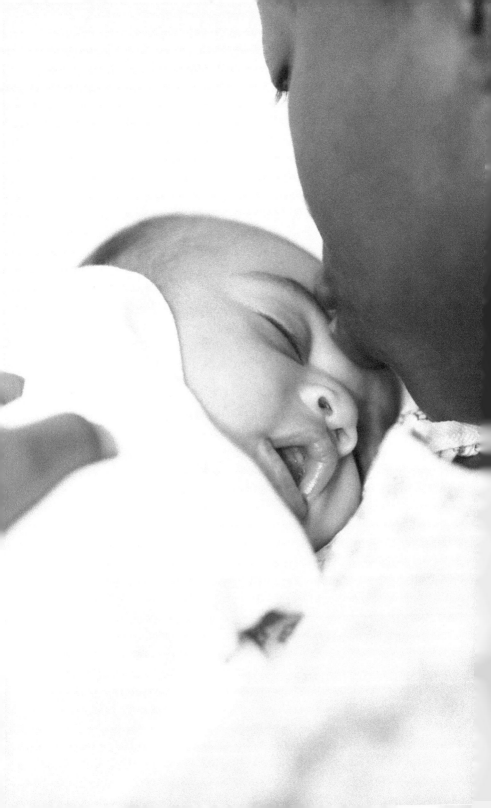

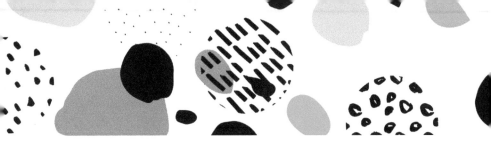

Resources

Websites

Evidence Based Birth (EvidenceBasedBirth.com) is an invaluable tool full of evidence-based, non-biased information for pregnant people. It also has a wonderful podcast.

Motherboard Birth (MotherboardBirth.com) is hands down the best resource I have seen to help families create birth plans.

Books

Reproductive Justice by **Loretta J. Ross and Rickie Solinger** is a powerful and important book that introduces the reader to the field of reproductive justice.

Reproductive Injustice by **Dána-Ain Davis** is a well-researched look at what it's like to be black and pregnant in America.

Organizations

The **American Association of Birth Centers** (AABC) is the national organization for birth centers. Its website (Birth Centers.org) is full of resources, including a "Find a Birth Center" tab.

The **American College of Nurse Midwives** (ACNM) is the national organization of certified nurse midwives. Its website

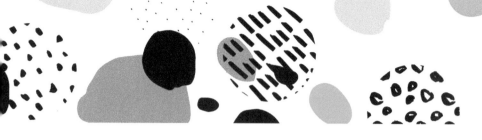

(Midwife.org) has a "Find a Midwife" tab as well many other resources for expectant parents.

Black Mamas Matter Alliance (BlackMamasMatter.org) is a group dedicated to decreasing the disparities and inequities for black woman and babies in America.

The **Changing Woman Initiative** (ChangingWoman Initiative.com) is, in the words of its mission statement, a "non-profit organization with the mission to renew cultural birth knowledge to empower and reclaim indigenous sovereignty of women's medicine."

Elephant Circle (ElephantCircle.net) is a birth justice organization dedicated to supporting consumers around reproductive rights issues.

The **National Association of Certified Professional Midwives** (NACPM) is the national organization for CPMs. Its website (NACPM.org) is full of resources and information for expectant parents.

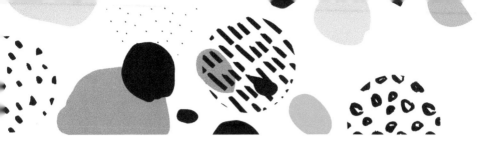

References

CHAPTER 1

American Association of Birth Centers. "New Government Report Recommends Birth Center Care." November 9, 2018. https://www.birthcenters.org/page/strong-start-report.

American College of Nurse-Midwives. "Midwifery: Evidence-Based Practice: A Summary of Research on Midwifery Practice in the United States." Last modified April 2012. https://www.midwife.org/acnm/files/ccLibraryFiles /Filename/000000004184/Midwifery-Evidence-Based -Practice-March-2013.pdf.

American College of Nurse-Midwives. "Our Philosophy of Care." Accessed February 28, 2020. https://www.midwife.org /Our-Philosophy-of-Care.

Bernitz, Stine, Pål Øian, Leiv Sandvik, and Ellen Blix. "Evaluation of Satisfaction with Care in a Midwifery Unit and an Obstetric Unit: A Randomized Controlled Trial of Low-Risk Women." *BMC Pregnancy Childbirth* 16, no. 1 (June 2016): 143. doi:10.1186/s12884-016-0932-x.

Ehrenreich, Barbara, and Deirdre English. *Witches, Midwives & Nurses: A History of Women Healers* (Second Edition). New York: The Feminist Press, 2010.

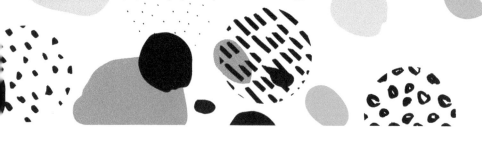

Emons, J. K., and M. I. J. Luiten. *Midwifery in Europe: An Inventory in Fifteen EU-Member States*. Bilthoven, The Netherlands: Deloitte & Touche, 2001.

Holtz-Carriere, Minnow. "Midwives." Women of Antiquity (blog). April 3, 2017. https://womeninantiquity.wordpress.com/2017/04/03/midwives.

International Confederation of Midwives. "Philosophy and Model of Midwifery Care." 2014. https://www.internationalmidwives.org/assets/files/definitions-files/2018/06/eng-philosophy-and-model-of-midwifery-care.pdf.

Kassebaum, Nicholas J., et al. "Global, Regional, and National Levels of Maternal Mortality, 1990–2015: A Systematic Analysis for the Global Burden of Disease Study 2015." *The Lancet* 388, no. 10053 (October 2016): 1775–812. doi:10.1016/S0140-6736(16)31470-2.

Manniën, Judith, et al. "Evaluation of Primary Care Midwifery in the Netherlands: Design and Rationale of a Dynamic Cohort Study." *BMC Health Services Research* 12, (March 2012): 69. doi:10.1186/1472-6963-12-69.

Maternal Health Task Force at the Harvard Chan School Center of Excellence in Maternal and Child Health. "Maternal Health in the United States." Accessed February

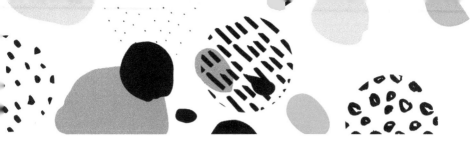

28, 2020. https://www.mhtf.org/topics/maternal-health-in-the
-united-states.

Mulder, Tara. "Midwifery in Modern China." Midwifery
around the World (blog). December 12, 2018. https://medium
.com/midwifery-around-the-world/midwifery-in-modern
-china-e6a8f51b5ee1.

Robinson, Karina. "Childbirth in Ancient Egypt: Nature's
Unique Work of Art." *Probe Magazine*. June 27, 2018.
https://www.ssbprobe.com/articles/childbirth-in-egypt.

Rochman, Bonnie. "Midwife Mania? More U.S. Babies Than
Ever Are Delivered by Midwives." *Time*. June 25, 2012.
https://healthland.time.com/2012/06/25/midwife-mania
-more-u-s-babies-than-ever-are-delivered-by-midwives.

Rooks, Judith P. "The History of Midwifery." Our Bodies,
Ourselves (website). Last modified May 22, 2014.
https://www.ourbodiesourselves.org/book-excerpts/health
-article/history-of-midwifery.

Scarlata, Miranda. "Midwifery in Japan." Midwifery around
the World (blog). December 11, 2018. https://medium
.com/midwifery-around-the-world/midwifery-in-japan
-6c2685748b70.

Stephenson, Jo. "Only Half of Babies in England Now
Delivered by Midwives." *Nursing Times*. November 15, 2016.

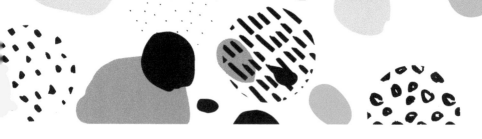

https://www.nursingtimes.net/news/hospital/only-half-of
-babies-in-england-now-delivered-by-midwives-15-11-2016.

Various authors. "Midwifery" (series). *The Lancet* (website). Last modified June 23, 2014. https://www.thelancet.com /series/midwifery.

Varney, Helen, and Joyce BeeBe Thompson. *A History of Midwifery in the United States: The Midwife Said Fear Not.* New York: Springer Publishing, 2016.

Vedam, Saraswathi, et al. "Mapping Integration of Midwives across the United States: Impact on Access, Equity, and Outcomes." *PLOS ONE* 13, no. 2 (February 2018): e0192523. doi:10.1371/journal.pone.0192523.

Wertz, Richard W., and Dorothy C. Wertz. *Lying-In: A History of Childbirth in America.* New York: Schocken Books, 1977.

CHAPTER 2

American Association of Birth Centers. "Position Statement: Immersion in Water during Labor and Birth." April 1, 2014. https://cdn.ymaws.com/www.birthcenters.org /resource/resmgr/about_aabc_-_documents/AABC_PS_-_ Immersion _in_Water.pdf.

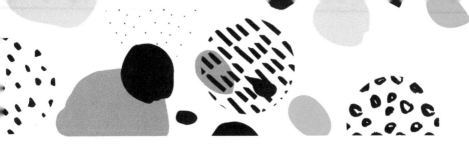

American Pregnancy Association. "Epidural Anesthesia." Last modified October 13, 2019. https://americanpregnancy .org/labor-and-birth/epidural.

Dekker, Rebecca. "Water Immersion during Labor for Pain Relief." Evidence-Based Birth (blog). April 3, 2018. https://evidencebasedbirth.com/water-immersion-during -labor-for-pain-relief.

Dunn, Alexis. B., Sheila Jordan, Brenda J. Baker, and Nicole S. Carlson. "The Maternal Infant Microbiome: Considerations for Labor and Birth." *The American Journal of Maternal/Child Nursing* 42, no. 6 (November 2017): 318–325. doi:10.1097/NMC.0000000000000373.

Jansen, Lauren, Martha Gibson, Betty Carlson Bowles, and Jane Leach. "First Do No Harm: Interventions during Childbirth." *The Journal of Perinatal Education* 22, no. 2. (Spring 2013): 83–92. doi:10.1891/1058-1243.22.2.83.

Keag, Oonagh, J. E. Norman, and S. J. Stock. "Long-Term Risks and Benefits Associated with Cesarean Delivery for Mother, Baby, and Subsequent Pregnancies: Systematic Review and Meta-Analysis." *PLoS Medicine* 15, no. 1. (January 2018): e1002494. doi:10.1371/journal.pmed.1002494.

Liu, Shiliang, et al. "Maternal Mortality and Severe Morbidity Associated with Low-Risk Planned Cesarean Delivery versus Planned Vaginal Delivery at Term."

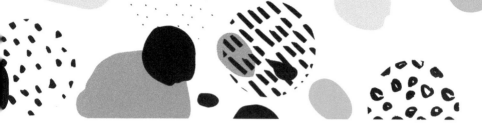

Canadian Medical Association Journal 176, no. 4 (February 13, 2007): 455–60. doi:10.1503/cmaj.060870.

McCarthy, Niall. "The U.S. Is the World's Most Expensive Nation for Childbirth." Forbes.com. January 29, 2020. https://www.forbes.com/sites/niallmccarthy/2020/01/29 /the-us-is-the-worlds-most-expensive-nation-for-childbirth -infographic/#1b2b0c12ec7f.

National Partnership for Women and Families. "The Cascade of Intervention." Childbirth Connection. Accessed February 28, 2020. http://www.childbirthconnection.org /maternity-care/cascade-of-intervention.

Nierenberg, Cari. "Vaginal Birth vs. C-Section: Pros & Cons." LiveScience. March 27, 2018. https://www.livescience .com/45681-vaginal-birth-vs-c-section.html.

Searing, Linda. "21 Percent of Babies Are Now Born by C-section, Nearly Double the Rate in 2000." The Big Number. *The Washington Post.* November 17, 2018. https: //www.washingtonpost.com/national/health-science/the-big -number--21-percent-of-babies-are-born-by-c-section-nearly -double-the-rate-in-2000/2018/11/16/ae539bfe-e8ef-11e8 -bbdb-72fdbf9d4fed_story.html.

Stapleton, Susan Rutledge, Cara Osborne, and Jessica Illuzzi. "Outcomes of Care in Birth Centers: Demonstration of a Durable Model." *Journal of Midwifery*

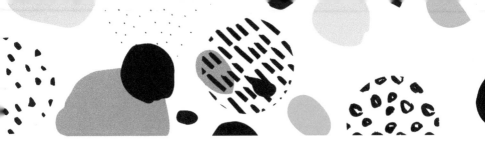

and Women's Health 58, no. 1 (January/February 2013): 13–14.
doi:10.1111/jmwh.12003.

White, Tracie. "Epidurals Increase in Popularity, Stanford
Study Finds." Scope by Stanford Medicine (blog). June 26,
2018. https://scopeblog.stanford.edu/2018/06/26/epidurals
-increase-in-popularity-stanford-study-finds.

CHAPTER 3

Mayo Clinic Staff. "Miscarriage." Mayo Clinic. Accessed
February 28, 2020. https://www.mayoclinic.org/diseases
-conditions/pregnancy-loss-miscarriage/symptoms-causes
/syc-20354298.

Varney, Helen, Jan M. Kriebs, and Carolyn L. Gegor.
Varney's Midwifery. 4th ed. Burlington: Jones and Bartlett,
2004.

CHAPTER 5

Chen, Er-mei, Meei-Ling Gau, Chieh-Yu Liu, and
Tzu-Ying Lee. "Effects of Father-Neonate Skin-to-Skin
Contact on Attachment: A Randomized Controlled Trial."
Nursing Research and Practice 2017 (2017): 8612024.
doi:10.1155/2017/8612024.

Crenshaw, Jeannette T. "Healthy Birth Practice #6: Keep
Mother and Baby Together—It's Best for Mother, Baby, and

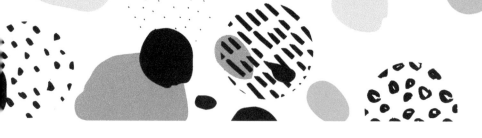

Breastfeeding." *The Journal of Perinatal Education* 23, no. 4 (Fall 2014): 211–17. doi:10.1891/1058-1243.23.4.211.

Haelle, Tara. "Delayed Umbilical Cord Clamping May Benefit Children Years Later." Shots: Health News from NPR. May 26, 2015. https://www.npr.org/sections/health -shots/2015/05/26/409697568/delayed-umbilical-cord -clamping-may-benefit-children-years-later.

Higuera, Valencia. "What Is a Birthing Ball and Should I Use One?" Healthline. Last updated November 18, 2019. https://www.healthline.com/health/pregnancy/what-is-a -birthing-ball-and-should-i-use-one.

Mercer, Judith S., et al. "Effects of Delayed Cord Clamping on 4-Month Ferritin Levels, Brain Myelin Content, and Neurodevelopment: A Randomized Controlled Trial." *The Journal of Pediatrics* 203 (December 2018): 266–72. doi:10.1016/j.jpeds.2018.06.006.

Stapleton, Susan Rutledge, Cara Osborne, and Jessica Illuzzi. "Outcomes of Care in Birth Centers: Demonstration of a Durable Model." *Journal of Midwifery and Women's Health* 58, no. 1 (January/February 2013): 13–14. doi:10.1111/jmwh.12003.

World Health Organization. *Guideline: Delayed Umbilical Cord Clamping for Improved Maternal and Infant Health and Nutrition Outcomes.* Geneva: World Health Organization, 2014. https://www.ncbi.nlm.nih.gov/books/NBK310514.

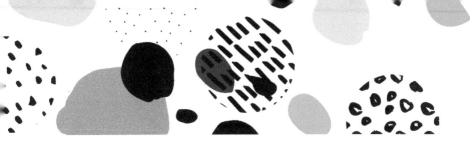

CHAPTER 6

American Academy of Pediatrics. "Safe Sleep." Accessed February 28, 2020. https://www.aap.org/en-us/advocacy-and -policy/aap-health-initiatives/healthy-child-care/Pages/Safe -Sleep.aspx.

American Academy of Pediatrics. "Benefits of Breastfeeding." Accessed February 28, 2020. https://www.aap.org/en-us/ advocacy-and-policy/aap-health-initiatives/Breastfeeding /Pages/Benefits-of-Breastfeeding.aspx.

National Institute of Mental Health. "Postpartum Depression Facts." Accessed February 28, 2020. https://www .nimh.nih.gov/health/publications/postpartum-depression -facts/index.shtml.

University of Notre Dame Mother-Baby Behavioral Sleep Laboratory. "Safe Cosleeping Guidelines." Accessed February 28, 2020. https://cosleeping.nd.edu/safe-co-sleeping -guidelines.

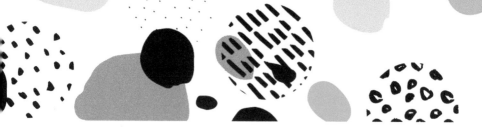

Wiessinger, Diane, Diana West, Linda J. Smith, and Teresa Pitman. "The Safe Sleep Seven." In *Sweet Sleep: Nighttime and Naptime Strategies for the Breastfeeding Family*, a La Leche League International book. New York: Ballantine Books, 2014. https://www.llli.org/the-safe-sleep-seven.

World Health Organization. "Breastfeeding." Accessed February 28, 2020. https://www.who.int/health-topics /breastfeeding#tab=tab_1.

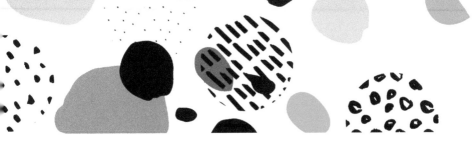

Index

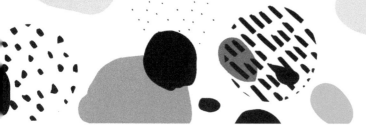
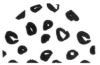

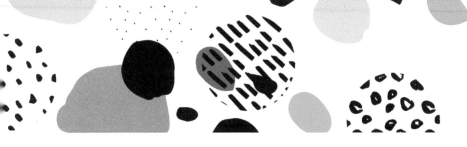

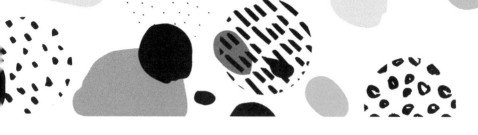

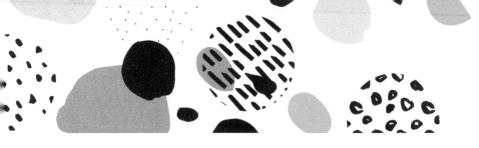

Acknowledgments

Writing this book has been a true labor of love and one that would not have been possible without the support of my community. I would first like to acknowledge that the land I live on, where I practice my midwifery, was colonized by my predecessors. It was originally inhabited by the Ute, Arapaho, Cheyenne, and Sioux. I would like to honor these peoples and give thanks to them and the land.

I am blessed to practice midwifery with a team of amazing folks, from midwives to nurses, physicians, researchers, medical assistants, and administrative experts. Without them, I would not have been able to craft this book. They are my second family, my resources, my support, and my home away from home.

Then, of course, there is my first family. My parents, who have always had an unstoppable faith in me and my dreams and have been my biggest cheerleaders. My husband and children, who are my heart and soul. Without any of these folks, I could not do what I do. I am thankful for each and every one of them.

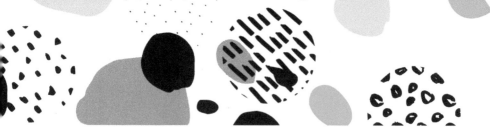

About the Author

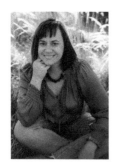

AUBRE TOMPKINS is a certified nurse midwife and director of midwifery at Seasons Midwifery & Birth Center in Colorado. She has been a midwife for over a decade and before that was a registered nurse in the obstetrical field for five years. Aubre is a faculty member for the American Association of Birth Centers, for which she travels the country teaching workshops about birth centers. She also serves on the board of directors of Birthwise Midwifery School in Maine.

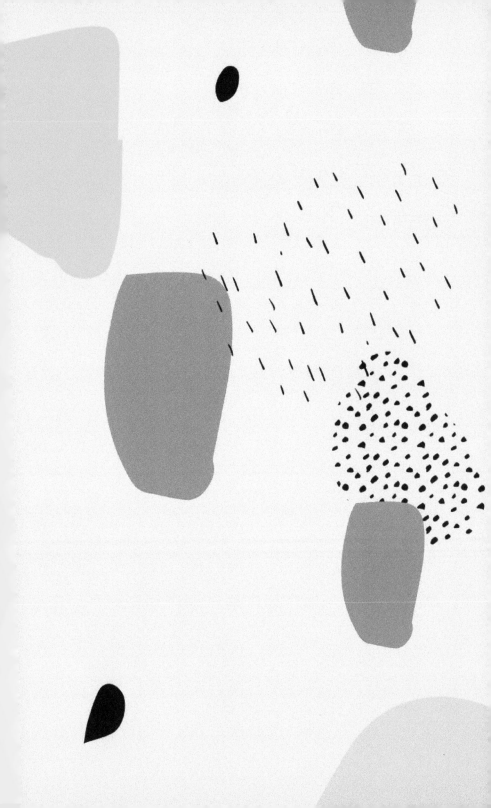